?

Exercise on Prescription:
Cardiovascular Activity for Health

Dedicated to: Trudy Buckley and all those who suffer from Alzheimer's disease. As a mother and a public health nurse she has always held high the ideal that good health and quality of life were more than the mere absence of illness. The virtues she extolled to her own children and those she nursed were that being healthy required a holistic combination of healthy eating, physical activity, quality rest, and the development of mental, social and spiritual well-being.

Exercise on Prescription: Cardiovascular Activity for Health

John Buckley BPE, MSc
Exercise Physiologist, Lifestyle Fitness, Shrewsbury; Research Fellow,
Department of Physiotherapy Studies, Keele University

Jane Holmes MCSP, MSc
Lecturer, Department of Physiotherapy Studies, Keele University

Gareth Mapp BA (Hons), MSc
Sports and Exercise Science Consultant, Lifestyle Fitness, Shrewsbury

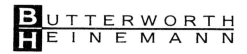

OXFORD AUCKLAND BOSTON JOHANNESBURG MELBOURNE NEW DELHI

Butterworth-Heinemann
Linacre House, Jordan Hill, Oxford OX2 8DP
225 Wildwood Avenue, Woburn, MA 01801-2041
A division of Reed Educational and Professional Publishing Ltd

ᴚ   A member of the Reed Elsevier plc group

First published 1999

British Library Cataloguing in Publication Data

A catalogue record for this book is available from the British Library

Library of Congress Cataloguing in Publication Data

A catalogue record for this book is available from the Library of Congress

ISBN 0 7506 3288 7

Printed and bound in Great Britain by Martins the Printers, Berwick upon Tweed

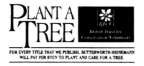

PLANT A TREE
FOR EVERY TITLE THAT WE PUBLISH, BUTTERWORTH-HEINEMANN
WILL PAY FOR BTCV TO PLANT AND CARE FOR A TREE

Contents

Preface   ix

1 Introduction: well-being, health, physical activity, exercise and fitness   1

Health-related versus sports-related fitness   3
The link between exercise, well-being and health   3
Thresholds for improved health and fitness from physical activity and
   exercise   4
References   8

2 The links between cardiovascular health, physical activity and exercise   11

An understanding of risk factors   12
Epidemiology, exercise and health in large populations   13
Beliefs and attitudes   15
How much activity is enough to modify the risk factors?   17
Discerning the difference: activity for health and exercise for fitness   18
Risk factor modification and exercise   19
References   26

3 Psychological aspects of physical activity and exercise   31

Part I Introduction to psychology and links with physical activity and exercise   32
Psychology, physical activity and exercise   33
Part II Exercise, physical activity and mental well-being   35
The cost and benefits   35
Negative psychological aspects of physical activity and exercise   43
How physical activity may improve mental health – the mechanisms   46
Part III Developing the 'exercise habit'   49
Adherence to exercise   49
Behaviour – cues and consequences   50
Barriers to exercise and physical activity participation   54
Beliefs and attitudes about physical activity and exercise   57
The process of changing exercise behaviour   58
Chapter summary   66
References   66

4   The science of aerobic exercise   71

A brief history   71
The science   75
References   88

5   The importance of understanding and acknowledging training status   91

Potential   91
Appreciating $\dot{V}O_{2max}$ only when considered alongside training status   93
References   94

6   Monitoring exercise responses: heart rate, ratings of perceived exertion and blood pressure   97

Heart rate   97
Ratings of perceived exertion   104
Blood pressure   112
References   113

7   Prescribing activity and exercise for health and fitness   115

What are people's activity choices?   116
Setting the intensity of activity – the key element   116
Increasing activity in daily living versus the traditional 'three times per week for 20 minutes' message   119
Performing daily activity tasks using ratings of perceived exertion and heart rate   124
Ensuring a clear understanding of the concept of exercise workrate   130
Establishing exercise workrates or target heart rates from ratings of perceived exertion during a submaximal exercise cycle text   131
Chapter summary   140
References   140

8   Protocols for predicting and estimating aerobic activity   141

Review of the protocols   141
Considerations for choosing the appropriate predictive $\dot{V}O_{2max}$ protocol   152
References   153

9 User friendly tables and charts for prescribing exercise with aerobic equipment 155

The physiological basis of exercise prescription intensities (pace) in relation to VO_{2max} and training status   155
User friendly charts for prescribing exercise intensities   157
Chapter summary   161
References   161

10 Muscle, bone and joint considerations for cardiovascular exercise 163

Responses and adaptations of the muscles, bones and joints (the musculo-skeletal system)   164
Preventing muscle, bone and joint problems in the newcomer   165
Acknowledging weight-bearing and non-weight-bearing modes of activity   166
Posture and the spine–lower limb interface during various aerobic activities   167

11 Activity and exercise considerations for high blood pressure and heart disease 179

Hypertension and associated health problems   181
Effects of beta blockers: implications for exercise   186
Considerations for those with coronary heart disease   190
Chapter summary   198
References   198

12 Health and exercise consultations 203

Measurements and changes   203
Setting the scene for the consultation   206
The consultation process   207
Part A. The subjective psychological, social, activity and medical history   207
Part B. The aims of the exercise programme for the client   219
Part C. Objective health and fitness measures   220
Part D. Cardiovascular fitness and the exercise programme and prescription   224
References   224

Index   225

Preface

This book is a culmination of theory, practice and experience of applied sports and exercise science which has essentially underpinned work being carried out in a real setting for over nine years. The original real setting for this work is the Lifestyle Fitness and Physiotherapy Centre located in the Shropshire county town of Shrewsbury, but as noted in the following paragraphs the application of this work has continued to spread and evolve to other 'arenas'.

The theoretical foundation of this book has been applied in the provision of over 4000 personalized exercise assessments, prescriptions and supervised programmes. This application more recently included the establishment of a new high-quality Exercise for Health Centre at the Royal Shrewsbury Hospital, which offers a three-tracked service intergrated into one facility. This integrated facility offers a corporate exercise centre for staff use, an exercise rehabilitation centre for cardiac patients and a centre to which community-based doctors can refer individuals for secondary preventative and health-promoting activity.

A key element to this book is the user friendly tables, which have been designed to eliminate many of the tedious calculations required to effectively measure fitness and establish beneficial exercise intensities. In reading through many exercise physiology texts and research papers, numerous mathematical models have been recommended for making such calculations, but there are essentially two inherent problems in using the calculations.

The first problem is that not all front-line exercise professionals are mathematically minded, and even though they may clearly understand the concept behind the calculations they find it somewhat 'off-putting' to have to collect data and then get their calculator out. Such calculations are often only easily usable by postgraduate level sports and exercise science academics, but these people are usually not on the front-line delivering the practice which is based on the theory. The second problem is that in a practical situation (i.e. a health and exercise assessment/consultation), time used in making calculations could be better spent on interacting with the client or patient. However, by having a set of tables it significantly reduces the time otherwise involved with using a pencil, paper and calculator. The exercise professional can produce the results much more easily and provide almost immediate feedback and guidance to the client or patient.

The need for these tables first arose when the personnel at the Lifestyle Fitness and Physiotherapy Centre were approached by the Oswestry School of Physiotherapy (this school is now based at Keele University in Staffordshire) to teach its students the application of exercise physiology for rehabilitative and health promotion based activity. From this point, the user friendly tables swiftly gained credence and not only did the students benefit but the practitioners at the Centre improved the quality of their service by using the tables on a day-to-day basis. Some of the tables and guidelines have recently been developed for the sake of improving the practicalities of using this book, and again this has been reflected back into the classroom for the students and into the consultation rooms for the practitioner. A further event has evolved as a result of bringing the practicalities of applying the theory in the consultation room into the physiotherapy classroom. The curriculum development in health-based exercise for physiotherapy students at Keele University has led to three first-time events in Britain. All three of these events, listed below, now form part of the the core undergraduate curriculum in the degree in physiotherapy offered at Keele University:

- For the first time, the exercise consultation room and the exercise centre gymnasium have become essentially another classroom for individual physiotherapy students attending a six-week clinical learning and training placement. Students are graded as in other clinical placements and this forms part of their final grade.
- For the first time in an undergraduate physiotherapy course, a university has accredited a full 12-week module in health-related exercise, where again the students are examined and given a grade.
- For the first time, physiotherapy students have been tutored on their clinical placement not by physiotherapists but by qualified exercise physiologists.

The authors of this book are those tutors and lecturers mentioned above. It is hoped that the inter-professional collaboration of this book, between exercise scientists and physiotherapists, continues in other institutions and is an example of how true multidisciplinary practice can be forged to provide optimal benefits both to clients and patients.

By no means, however, should this book be thought of as a comprehensive exercise science text such as those written by Astrand and Rodahl, McArdle and Katch, and Costill and Wilmore. It has the specific aim to be a supplementary practical guide for prescribing cardiovascular/aerobic activity 'on the front line' with real clients. It is also designed for use within exercise educational training programmes, whether they are university based courses or vocational courses like those offered at community/technical colleges or the YMCA.

Although it may seem rather contrived and coincidental, the authors feel it is very fitting for the development of this book to have occurred in Shropshire, a country which has had a significant impact on the industrialization and hence the sedentary lifestyle of the Western world, on the modern Olympic games, and on medical science. Key elements related to these three factors are the main thrust behind the information contained in this book.

The town of Ironbridge near Telford, Shropshire, is the birthplace of the Industrial Revolution, which also means the birthplace of our modern mechanized and consequently sedentary Western society. It is the advances of modern engineering and technology, arising from the Industrial Revolution, that have unfortunately contributed to the Western world becoming far more sedentary than those of our ancestors whose daily occupations involved direct physical labour for obtaining food, water and shelter. Many of our more serious chronic and acute contemporary health concerns (i.e. heart disease, hypertension and acquired diabetes) are directly related to a sedentary lifestyle, which will be highlighted in the first two chapters. It is of interest to have found two books, written before 1910, in a second-hand bookshop in Iron-bridge, warning readers of the potential effects of sedentary living. The first book was a 1909 English Education Authority's Syllabus for teaching physical education; even then, it was mentioned that one of the prime needs of regular physical exercise was to ward off the effects of sedentary living. The second book was a 1907 manual of human physiology by Leonard Hill, in which he stated:

There is no lesson which more needs to be learnt by man, for it was known by the ancient Greeks: healthy mental development cannot advance without muscular development. Let the indolent women and the hard work sempstress scrub floors and the lazy man or hard-worked scholar dig the ground for two hours a day and half the medical profession would starve for lack of patients

The research referred to throughout this book will no doubt qualify the above comments with an uncanny similarity.

So much of the study of human performance and sport and exercise science which underpins the theory in this book has come about through the fascination of scientists studying athletes of modern Olympic calibre. Although many are aware that Baron Pierre de Coubertin was the Father of the modern Olympics, much of his inspiration came from Dr William Penny Brookes. Brookes, in the small Shropshire town of Much Wenlock, was organising what he actually called Olympic Games for 40 years prior to the first modern Olympics of 1896. It is well documented how de Coubertin visited and consulted Brookes on the setting up of the modern Olympic movement.

Finally, medical and human science has gained so much from Charles Darwin, who was born and educated in Shrewsbury. His concept of natural selection and (commonly referred to as the survival of the fittest) could not be more appropriate to the need for health-related exercise/activity. It is unfortunate that some people are born with genes that may predispose them to cardiovascular disease. Compound this problem with a stressful sedentary lifestyle and the risk of heart disease is greatly increased. A healthy active lifestyle can actually ward off the effects of inherited risks towards heart disease, as continually noted throughout the early chapters, and thus in spite of poor 'natural selection' of a set of parents, an increase in daily activity can prevent or at least delay the onset of a serious heart attack. It must be accepted, though seemingly unfair, that there are those who have 'naturally selected' good parents and the potential to achieve physical success gives them an even better chance towards survival of the fittest.

Chapters 1–6 provide the necessary theoretical information which it is essential to understand fully before the activity and exercise prescription guidelines given in Chapter 7 onwards are adopted.

Another main aim of this book is that it focuses on using facts and figures, calculated with the user-friendly tables, as prescriptive data as opposed to merely descriptive information about a client's state of health or fitness. For example, one of the most common elements of an exercise assessment is the determination or estimation of maximal aerobic capacity ($\dot{V}O_{2max}$). Many courses of instruction within the health and fitness industry merely use $\dot{V}O_{2max}$ to describe where an individual stands (often as a percentile) in relation to the general population, rather than using it as a basis of prescription. Does the client really understand what a score of $\dot{V}O_{2max}$ means? It is now known that 70–80% of Western populations are inactive (expend less than 20 000 cal per week), as shown by large-scale studies in Britain, Canada and the USA. There is thus a high probability that anyone starting exercise from a sedentary state is likely to have a poor rating or percentile ranking, and that assessment results, if used improperly, only confirm what the client already knows.

The final chapter, on the exercise consultation, addresses more importantly how the client feels and why they 'want' or 'need' to become more physically active. It addresses the client's needs and the psychological and social barriers which may affect their participation. This final chapter focuses on how to take a positive approach to getting clients to accept any physical, social or psychological perceived restraints and that any participation and improvement, no matter how large or small, is a step towards better health.

A very important point to remember is that the scientific basis of exercise assessments and prescriptions is not an end in itself. It is the application of this information, which is a tool for encouraging people to modify their lifestyle behaviour and state of well-being. The numbers and scores an exercise professional/clinician collects, as stated previously are often meaningless to the client or patient. What is important to the client is that you have helped them, by effective guidance, prescription and instruction, to be aware of indicators that their health and behaviour have changed or improved. The guidelines and tables are designed to be used on a daily basis with each and every consultation, whether for a new client or a follow-up re-evaluation.

Acknowledgements

The authors would like to thank: **Christine Jennings** and **Alan Leigh** (Chartered Physiotherapists), partners of the Lifestyle Fitness and Physiotherapy Centre, Shrewsbury, for their high level of involvement over the past nine years in helping deliver, 'on the front-line', the principles found within the pages of this book. **Tracey Heron** for her assistance in writing Chapter 10. **All the exercise instructors at both the Lifestyle and Shrewsbury Hospital exercise centres** for being at the 'sharp end' of administering and motivating clients receiving the potential benefits discussed in this book. **Marilyn Place** for supporting and encouraging the academic principles within this book as part of pioneering efforts in bridging the 'perceived' gap between the traditional concepts of *physiotherapy* and more contemporary ideals of *movement and exercise science*. **The thousands of clients and patients of the Lifestyle and Shrewsbury Hospital exercise centres**, for whom without their trust in the authors' efforts and all those mentioned above provide a 'soul' to the meaning of the pages to follow.

1

Introduction: well-being, health, physical activity, exercise and fitness

Health-related versus sports-related fitness
The link between exercise, well-being and health
Thresholds for improved health and fitness from physical activity and
  exercise
References

Within the media and the literature the terms *well-being, health, physical activity, exercise* and *fitness* are often interlinked and possibly used interchangeably. Yet these terms each have specific definitions, which should be used appropriately. In the next few paragraphs a brief definition of each term will be given, followed by further elaboration.

Health and well-being are more than just the absence of illness, but terms which encompass the combined state of four elements:[1,2]

- physical health,
- mental health,
- social health,
- spiritual health.

A person who has a good level of well-being is physically, mentally, socially and spiritually healthy all at the same time (Figure 1.1), something quite difficult to achieve! The concept of a health continuum, ranging from complete illness to high-level well-being will be described and illustrated in Chapter 3.

Physical activity is any voluntary muscle movement or action which raises the energy demands of the body and the rate of blood circulation above that of a resting state. Even performing domestic chores and gardening can be included as physical activities. It is often heard that some individuals live a physically active life which includes both their home life and their work (the farmer, the postman who walks or uses a

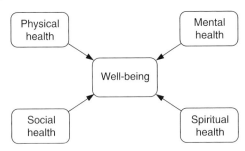

Figure 1.1 Factors contributing to well-being. (Adapted from the WHO Constitution[1] and Grant *et al.*[2])

bicycle, or a construction worker). Two notable studies which have looked at the health status of workers based on the amount of physical activity during work are: the London bus conductor versus driver study[3] and the longshoreman study.[4]

Both studies showed that those with more active jobs had a lower incidence of heart disease and related health risk factors. With the advancement of machinery and technology in the last century, life especially in the industrialized world has become much less physically active.

The acknowledgement of the effects of low levels of daily physical activity on health have led to the popular concept in the last 200 years, of structured leisure time physical activity known as exercise. Exercise thus requires the intent to be physically active within a framework of time. Time has to be set aside to perform exercise and time is often used as one of the factors in measuring the performance of exercise capacity. The Earl of Derby once stated that 'those who cannot find time for bodily exercise will sooner or later have to find time for illness'. Exercise capacity can be given a rating, which is defined as fitness. The American College of Sports Medicine defines fitness 'as the ability to perform moderate to vigorous levels of physical activity without undue fatigue and the capability of maintaining such ability throughout life'.[5] Fitness is influenced by a number of attributes that people have or can achieve, including genetic make-up, general physical health and how much physical activity and exercise they regularly perform.[6,7] There are typically four elements of fitness:

- cardiovascular endurance,
- muscular endurance,
- muscular strength,
- flexibility of muscles and joints.

Fitness is also a historical concept associated with preparation for sending men off to war or battle. Training regimens were set up to improve endurance, strength and mobility for the requirements of battle. Today, many consider that exercise prepares them physically and mentally for the stresses of modern daily life. One of the biggest 'battles' now, dealt with in Chapter 2, is combating the unhealthy effects of sedentary living which are increasing in modern mechanized societies.

Metabolic fitness? The possible new fifth component

In May 1997 the American College of Sports Medicine discussed elements of a new 'Position Statement' on fitness training which included a new component called 'metabolic' fitness. This component included many of the blood and muscle chemical changes which occur as a result of increased activity and exercise training, including changes in cholesterol, responses to lactic acid, increased energy storage of muscle and reduced insulin resistance. Some of these changes may not manifest themselves in noticeable levels of improved 'overt' exercise performance, but may be important towards improved health (i.e. cholesterol changes and control or prevention of diabetes). The sections to follow in this chapter will look at both the health- and performance-related elements of fitness.

Health-related versus sports-related fitness

Improving fitness for health and well-being should incorporate all of the four elements of fitness above. From the perspective of this book, the main focus is cardiovascular endurance, which is closely associated with cardiovascular health. Chapter 2 highlights why cardiovascular fitness is so important as the keystone of health-based fitness. With regards to strength and joint flexibility, these too are important in performing daily functional activities (housework, gardening, moving objects or carrying). Life for people without basic strength and endurance, especially in the elderly, can be very debilitating by their having to be dependent on others.

Fitness for sports is typically much more specific to one of the four individual elements of fitness, depending on the nature of the sport – whether it requires strength and power (sprinting, throwing, hitting) or endurance (maintaining running speed for extended periods). Pursuing fitness for a specific physical goal or performance, whether against others or a stopwatch, can also reach a point where it is of no further benefit and possibly even a detriment to one's physical, mental and social health (see Figure 1.3, page 7).

The exercise professional needs to build up a profile of a client's or athlete's needs in order to prescribe the correct mixture of the four basic elements of fitness.

The link between exercise, well-being and health

Exercise, unlike most other health interventions, has the potential to benefit all the elements of well-being (physical, mental, social and spiritual). Beyond the physical benefits, exercise is closely allied to its influence on people's mental state and Chapter 3 will specifically look at this element. Exercise has also been acknowledged, in cases of health rehabilitation, with improving such conditions as high blood pressure[8–10] and postively affecting some mental illnesses.[11] By influencing one's physical and mental health, the act of participating in exercise can lead to improved social health, which is the ability to relate and interact with others, including family, friends and colleagues at work.[12] Exercise, by its nature, can create an arena for social interaction, which in itself can be beneficial.[13,14] In the right environment, exercise can possibly act as a social leveller for people regardless of their race, religion and socio-economic status.

Spiritual health acknowledges a person's level of happiness, from peace of mind to one's level of acceptance of the physical and social world around them. Many of the Eastern and Asian physical exercises and sports are intertwined with a spiritual ideal, belief or philosophy (e.g. Tai Chi, Judo, Karate, Sumo wrestling, Kung Fu). In Western society, physical activity, exercise and sport have been used as a social catalyst within spiritual retreats or gatherings, the most well-known of the twentieth century being the YMCA and YWCA (Young Men's/ Women's Christian Association). The YMCA has now evolved far beyond its original idea as a venue for social and spiritual respite, but has certainly left its mark as a great institution of physical recreation for developing the ideal of a 'sound body and sound mind'. Thomas Arnold, Headmaster of Rugby School in the mid-1800s, went to the length of coining the term 'muscular Christianity', to describe that sport and exercise were not just good for the body but good for the minds and attitudes (spirit) of young men.

Whatever one's beliefs, philosophies or attitudes, exercise and physical activity have a potential influence across all the four elements of health and well-being.

Thresholds for improved health and fitness from physical activity and exercise

It is now known that even low but regular levels of increased physical activity can help improve health, with benefits to blood pressure, cholesterol, weight and mental state.[15,16] It is possible to achieve health benefits by initiating more physcial activity into one's daily life, including:

- walking as a means of local transport as opposed to using the car or bus,
- walking the children to school rather than driving,
- using a bicycle as a means of transport.

Such increased physical activity may not result in large improvements in noticeable fitness, but even the few extra calories 'burned up' and increased circulation to the muscles can affect cholesterol, blood pressure and mental health, to a level which can lower the risks or at least control future health problems (diabetes, heart disease, stroke). In Chapter 2 the broader scale of the above health concerns will be addressed on how the general health of large populations are influenced by exercise and physical activity. Figure 1.2 from the US Surgeon General's Report outlines examples of moderate amounts of physical activity. Pursuing physical activity to higher levels of intensity may take on elements more suitable to be considered structured exercise training, at which a threshold is reached where measurable fitness improvements, in addition to health benefits, occur.[5]

Figure 1.3 illustrates that as a person increases the level of activity and exercise there are corresponding levels of improved health benefits. At an intensity which is about 50% of a person's aerobic capacity (VO_{2max}), fitness improvements can clearly be measured.[5] The recommended threshold for health and fitness benefits are at present being reviewed. A verbal report from Dr Michael Pollock, on behalf the American College of Sports Medicine, has suggested accepting a threshold as low as 40% of VO_{2max} for conferring some benefit in sedentary individuals. The amount of activity recommended is an accumulation of up to 30 minutes of physical activity per day, with minimum bouts of 10 minutes or more vigorous activity three times per week for 20 minutes. Chapter 2 will more fully outline the specific health benefits.

In addition to the health benefits of regular physical activity already described, regular aerobic exercise confers other health improvements, including:

- improvements in cardiac function,[17,18]
- maintenance of functional capacity (physical independence) in old age,[19,20]
- reducing depression,[21]
- possibly even the treatment and prevention of cancer.[22]

There comes a point, however, where general health benefits plateau and then some aspects of health may even decline with the specific desire to attain very high levels of fitness. In the Preface to a book called 'The Runner',[23] Sir Roger Bannister wrote about the running boom: 'for some almost an addiction, but if so the only healthy addiction I know.' Following on from Sir Roger's quote, it is interesting to note that psychologists have actually classified the addiction to exercise into either a positive healthy addiction[24] or a negative addiction.[25] With regards to the negative addiction, studies included not just the effects on physical health, where people continued training in spite of an injury, but also on the decline in social health affecting family life, relationships and lowered standards at work. Numerous studies have investigated the effects of high volumes of exercise training on many other health problems, including:

- anaemia,[26]
- infertility,[27]
- overuse stress fractures and soft tissue damage in the legs and arms,[28,29]
- reduced immunity and tolerance to both minor and major illnesses,[30,31]
- ultra endurance training damage to the heart.[32]

What is a moderate amount of physical activity?

As the examples listed in the box show, a moderate amount of physical activity* can be achieved in a variety of ways. People can select activities that they enjoy and that fit into their daily lives. Because amount of activity is a function of duration, intensity, and frequency, the same amount of activity can be obtained in longer sessions of moderately intense activities (such as brisk walking) as in shorter sessions of more strenuous activities (such as running):[†]

Examples of moderate amounts of activity

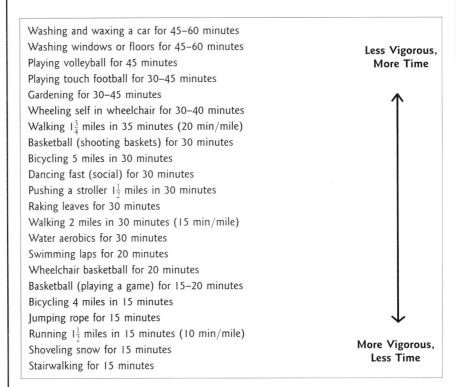

Washing and waxing a car for 45–60 minutes
Washing windows or floors for 45–60 minutes
Playing volleyball for 45 minutes
Playing touch football for 30–45 minutes
Gardening for 30–45 minutes
Wheeling self in wheelchair for 30–40 minutes
Walking $1\frac{3}{4}$ miles in 35 minutes (20 min/mile)
Basketball (shooting baskets) for 30 minutes
Bicycling 5 miles in 30 minutes
Dancing fast (social) for 30 minutes
Pushing a stroller $1\frac{1}{2}$ miles in 30 minutes
Raking leaves for 30 minutes
Walking 2 miles in 30 minutes (15 min/mile)
Water aerobics for 30 minutes
Swimming laps for 20 minutes
Wheelchair basketball for 20 minutes
Basketball (playing a game) for 15–20 minutes
Bicycling 4 miles in 15 minutes
Jumping rope for 15 minutes
Running $1\frac{1}{2}$ miles in 15 minutes (10 min/mile)
Shoveling snow for 15 minutes
Stairwalking for 15 minutes

Less Vigorous, More Time

More Vigorous, Less Time

*A moderate amount of physical activity is roughly equivalent to physical activity that uses approximately 150 calories of energy per day, or 1000 calories per week. [†] Some activities can be performed at various intensities; the suggested durations correspond to expected intensity of effort.

Precautions for a healthy start

To avoid soreness and injury, individuals contemplating an increase in physical activity should start out slowly and gradually build up to the desired amount to give the body time to adjust. People with chronic health problems, such as heart disease, diabetes, or obesity, or who are at high risk for these problems should first consult a physician before beginning a new program of physical activity. Also, men over age 40 and women over age 50 who plan to begin a new *vigorous* physical activity program should consult a physician first to be sure they do not have heart disease or other health problems.

Figure 1.2 US Surgeon General's Report summary on moderate amounts of physical activity (1996).

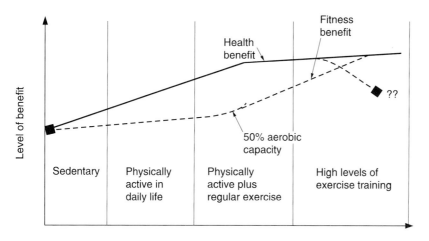

Figure 1.3 Levels of health and fitness benefit from increased amounts of physical activity and exercise. ?? = potential physical, social and psychosocial detriment of overtraining. (Adapted from the ACSM Position Stand[5] and the US Surgeon General's Report on health and physical activity, 1996.)

From Figure 1.3 and the corresponding points above, the cliché 'too much of a good thing can be bad for you' appears to be confirmed.

With the above clarification of the terms well-being, health, physical activity, exercise and fitness, the reader should now have good grounding for reading the following chapters.

A case report from the authors' experience, given below, illustrates the importance of how an exercise professional may need to be aware of the client's needs and potential desires, so that guidance can be given on ensuring a good balance between personal achievement social acceptance and the numerous parameters of physical health (both positive and negative) affected by exercise.

Case report

In working with members of the local road-running club, it is often typical for them to rise to the challenge of running the London Marathon. The aim often is both for the personal challenge and raising money for a charity. There is, however, an increased incidence of physical injury and family or social tension as more time is devoted to the training programme. Initially a person may join the running club for both social reasons and to get a little bit healthier and fitter. Over time a sense of personal achievement is gained, as measured by the ability to run a distance in excess of 10 km or completing a course in a certain time. The infamous 'personal best' or 'PB' is thus established and encouragement from other members of the club to do better soon follows. The personal challenge thus starts to grow and there is a new aim; to run further and faster, surpassing previous PBs, where the original objectives of joining the club (social contact and improved health and fitness) may start to be forgotten. A typical example of achievement, within a 6–8 month period of joining a running club, is completing about 20 miles per week along with the corresponding health benefits (weight loss, stamina and self-esteem). To this level the person has avoided any excess overuse injury and has not required too much time commitment away from existing social, family and work obligations. The profile of the person is one who was not necessarily successful at sport while at school, but is now between the ages of 35 and 50 and realising they can gain a feeling of physical success. However, both mechanically (as demonstrated by the abnormal wear on the sole of their running shoes) and physically (the capacity to sustain a running pace at best between 8–10 min per mile), the person has a higher chance of injury as compared to someone under the age of 30. The desire and challenge to run a marathon, however, overrides some common sense and thus more time away from the person's normal life will now be required. The person with lower levels of genetically determined fitness and mechanical muscle and bone design faults will require more time than the more gifted runner in order to meet the same mileage training targets for a marathon, which is 12–18 miles per session, aggregating to more than 30–45 miles per week. This is far beyond the minimum recommended quality and quantity of training necessary for health and fitness as outlined by the American College of Sports Medicine.[5] It is therefore important, when planning to train for events similar to a marathon or a triathlon, to acknowledge that the aim is a personal challenge, which goes far beyond the requirements for improved health. Careful planning must include both the physical and psychosocial limitations of each person. On an opposing note, it is somewhat impressive to hear about the cardiac rehabilitation patients of Dr Kavanagh in Toronto, who have gone from feelings of desperation and lack of self-esteem following their heart attack, to completing the New York Marathon. These patients, through their exercise, have regained a great sense of self-confidence that positively affects other aspects of their life and clearly demonstrates that it's never too late!

Chapter 3 further explores the reasons why people may behave as they do in the above case report. The possibilities could include an addiction to running, a refusal to accept the passage of time and attempting to retain their youth, something positive which counterbalances an unhappiness in other elements of their life at work or at home, or some other social obsession linked to the security of being accepted as a member of a club or group.

References

1. World Health Organisation Constitution (1947) *Chronicle 1*, WHO, Geneva, p. 29.
2. Grant, M., Ferre, B., Schmidt, G.M., Fonbuena, P. *et al.* (1992) Measurement of quality of life in bone marrow transplant survivors. *Qual. Life Res.*, **1**, 185–193.
3. Morris, J.N., Pattison, D.C., Kagan, A. and Gardner, M.J. (1966) Incidence and prediction of ischaemic heart disease in London busmen. *Lancet*, 10 Sep. **2**, 553–559.
4. Paffenbarger, R.S., Laughlin, M.E., Gima, A.S. *et al.* (1970) Work activity of longshoremen as related to death from coronary heart disease and stroke. *New Eng. J. Med.*, **282**, 1109–1114.
5. American College of Sports Medicine (1990) Position Stand: The recommended quantity and quality of exercise for developing and maintaining

cardiorespiratory and muscular fitness in healthy adults. *Med. Sci. Sports. Exerc.*, **22**(2), 265–274.

6. Astrand, P.O. and Rodahl, K. (1986) *Textbook of Work Physiology: Physiological Basis of Exercise*, McGraw-Hall, New York.

7. McArdle, W.D., Katch, F.I. and Katch, V.L. (1981) *Exercise Physiology– Energy Nutrition and Human Performance*, Lea and Ferbiger, New York.

8. Montoye, H.J., Metzner, H.L. and Keller, J.B. (1972) Habitual physical activity and blood pressure. *Med. Sci. Sports. Exerc.*, **4**, 175–181.

9. Nelson, L., Esler, M.D., Jennings, G.L. and Korner, P.I. (1986) Effect of changing levels of physical activity on blood pressure and haemodynamics in essential hypertension. *Lancet*, **2**, 473–476.

10. Somer, V.K., Conway, J., Johnston, J. *et al.* (1991) Effects of endurance training on baroreflex sensitivity and blood pressure in border-line hypertension. *Lancet*, **337**, 8754.

11. Weyerer, S. and Kupfer, B. (1994) Physical exercise and psychological health. *Sports Med.*, **17**(2), 108–116.

12. Fallowfield, L. (1990) *The Quality of Life. The Missing Measurement in Health Care*, Souvenir Press, London.

13. Janoski, M.L., Holmes, D.S., Solomon, S. and Aguir, C. (1981) Exercise changes in aerobic capacity and changes in self perception: an experimental investigation. *J. Personal. Res.*, **15**, 460–466.

14. King, A.C., Taylor, C.B., Haskell, W.L. and Debusk, R.F. (1989) Influence of regular aerobic exercise on psychological health: a randomised controlled trial of healthy middle-aged adults: *Health. Psychol.*, **8**, 305–324.

15. Davison, R.C.R. and Grant, S. (1993) Is walking sufficient exercise for health? *Sports Med.*, **16**(6), 369–373.

16. Hardman, A.E. and Hudson, A. (1989) Walking for health – a closer look at exercise. *Health Trends* (UK Dept. of Health), **3**, 21.

17. Donald, K.W., Bishop, J.M., Cumming, C. *et al.* (1955) The effect of exercise on the cardiac output and central dynamics of normal subjects. *Clinic. Sci.*, **14**, 37–73.

18. Morris, C.K. and Froelicher, V.F. (1993) Cardiovascular benefits of improved exercise capacity. *Sports Med.*, **16**(4), 225–236.

19. Green, J.S. and Crouse, S.F. (1993) Endurance training, cardiovascular function and the aged. *Sports Med.*, **16**(5), 331–341.

20. Young, A., Grieg, C., Parrt-Billings, M. and Newsholme, E.A. (1992) Strength and Power/Aerobic exercise. In *Oxford Textbook of Geriatric Medicine* (Evans, J.G and Williams, T.F., eds), Oxford University Press, Section 19, pp. 596–613.

21. McCann, L. and Holmes, D.S. (1984) Influence of aerobic exercise on depression. *J. Personality Soc. Psychol.*, **46**(5), 1142–1147.

22. Shephard, R.J. (1993) Exercise in the treatment and prevention of cancer: an update. *Sports Med.*, **15**(4), 258–280.

23. Newsolme, E. and Leech, T. (1985) *The Runner*, Walter L. Meager, Oxford.

24. Glasser, W. (1976) *Positive Addiction*, Harper and Row, New York.

25. Morgan, W.P. (1979) Negative addiction in runners. *Physician Sportsmed*, **7**, 57–70.

26. Smith, J.A. (1995). Exercise and red blood cell turnover. *Sports Med.*, **19**(1), 9–31.

27. Arce, J.C. and DeSouza, J.M. (1993) Exercise and male factor infertility. *Sports Med.*, **15**(3), 146–169.

28. Black, K.P. and Taylor, D.E. (1993) Current concepts in the treatment of common compartment syndromes. *Sports Med.*, **15**(6), 408–418.

29. van Mechelen, W. (1995) Can running injuries be effectively prevented. *Sports Med.*, **19**(6), 161–165.
30. Brenner, K., Shek, P.N. and Shephard, R. (1994) Infection in athletes. *Sports Med.*, **17**(2), 86–107.
31. Shephard, R.J. and Shek, P.N. (1993) Infection and the athlete. *Clin. J. Sports. Med.*, **3**, 57–77.
32. Rowe, W. (1993) Endurance exercise and injury to the heart. *Sports Med.*, **16**(2), 73–79.

2

The links between cardiovascular health, physical activity and exercise

An understanding of risk factors
Epidemiology, exercise and health in large populations
Beliefs and attitudes
How much activity is enough to modify the risk factors?
Discerning the difference: activity for health and exercise for fitness
Risk factor modification and exercise
References

Coronary heart disease (CHD), a condition characterized by a restriction in blood flow to the heart muscle and cerebrovascular accident or stroke (CVA), where blood flow to part of the brain has been restricted or has haemorrhaged, are the primary causes of premature death in Western, industrialized societies.[1] As the links between activity, exercise and cardiovascular health have now been established from research over the past four decades, it was felt that this topic merited a chapter of its own.

In Chapter 1 it was outlined that increased levels of regular physical activity and exercise were linked to a number of health benefits. Alongside cigarette smoking and poor diet, lack of physical activity has now been identified as one of the main behavioural contributors of CHD and CVA.[2–10] Lack of physical activity has also been shown to have an impact on many other risk factors which often lead to CHD and CVA, including obesity, diabetes, high blood pressure, and increased blood fibrinogen and cholesterol levels. All these CHD and CVA risk factors are discussed individually in this chapter.

Risk factors are defined as health conditions which have clearly been demonstrated to have a link with a particular disease. People who possess one or more of the risk factors noted above are more likely to have a greater chance of developing CHD or suffering a CVA.

An understanding of risk factors

There are two ways of classifying risk factors:[11,12]

- those which can be changed or modified (i.e. diet, cigarette smoking, exercises, drug therapy),
- those which cannot be modified (i.e. genetics, age, gender).

Figure 2.1 summarizes many of the CHD and CVA risk factors (see also accompanying sketch).

Research shows that CHD and CVA often arise from a whole 'cocktail' of these genetic and behavioural events[11,12] including:

- family history,
- smoking,
- lack of physical activity,
- being overweight and obesity,
- psychological and social stress.

It must be appreciated that it is difficult to determine precisely the contributing proportions of family history, genetics and behavioural

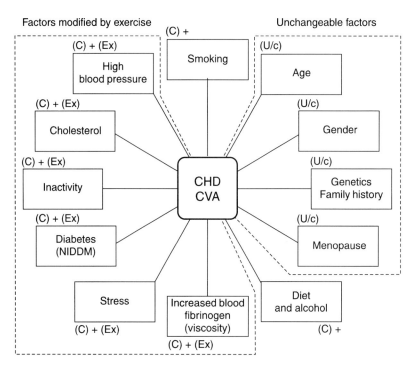

Figure 2.1 Associated risk factors for CHD and CVA (U/c, unchangeable or unmodifiable; C, changeable or modifiable through lifestyle changes; Ex, exercise has a beneficial effect on this risk factor). (Adapted from Wilmore and Costill[11] and Pollock and Schmidt.[12])

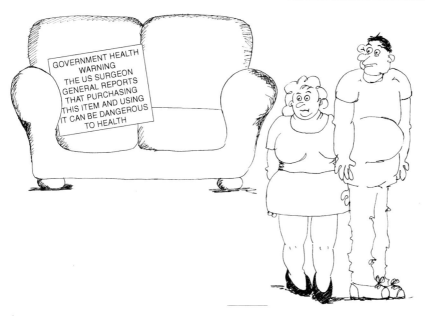

causes of CHD and CVA. Not only can a person inherit from their parents or grandparents the physical and chemical genetically-based disorders that predispose an individual to CHD or CVA, but one may also inherit the psychological characteristics and adopt social attitudes which can influence health behaviour.

Epidemiology, exercise and health in large populations

Epidemiology is the study of the nature and cause of disease in large populations. Research of this type has highlighted the link between health risk factors and the nature and cause of disease in large populations. In the 1950s, the first major studies into linking CHD and CVA with a lack of activity and exercise were undertaken with large numbers of subjects.[5,13] Some of these long-term studies have been continuing over many decades, and some are still in progress and continue to provide much up-to-date information alongside short-term studies. For epidemiological studies to be valid, Powell and Blair[7] have stated that a direct link must be shown between behaviour and disease and fulfil the following criteria:

- there must be consistency of relationship (inactive lifestyle and obesity),
- exposure to a risk factor precedes a disease outcome (smoking and lung cancer),
- there is a dose response (higher exposure leads to higher risk, i.e. less activity or more smoking increases the chances of having a heart attack),
- credibility; there must be a plausible and consistent relationship

within current knowledge, where numerous independent pieces of research have agreement,

- there must be a strong and persuasive relationship.

There is also the question of how long it will take before the risk of a disease is reduced following a change in lifestyle behaviour. Research has shown that risk reduction for CHD will progressively improve 2–3 years after cessation of smoking[14] and in a similar length of time following the commencement of regular physical activity.[7]

An overview of specific research studies now follows in the various sections of this chapter, which explore more fully the relationships between lifestyle behaviours and risk factors for CHD and CVA.

Main findings of the research

There have been a number of common findings from studies which have given credibility to the fundamental rationale of promoting exercise for health gains:

1. *The protective effect* of regular physical activity against the incidence of, and mortality from CHD.[2,4,5]
2. *There is a 50% reduction in CHD* in middle-aged to elderly men who have regularly participated in exercise all their lives.[6]
3. *A sedentary individual* is three times as likely to die early from CVA than a regularly active person.[15]
4. *Simple regular activity* (not necessarily sport) equivalent to a daily 20–30 minute brisk walk can be beneficial to health.[16] If the duration is greater than 30 minutes per day and the intensity of the exercise undertaken increases to a range of 40–70% of an individual's aerobic capacity, the protection against CHD is further increased.[4,17–21]
5. *It is never too late* to commence regular activity. Even when CHD risk factors have been identified or diagnosed and even after an MI (myocardial infarction or heart attack, where a blockage of blood flow to the heart muscle has caused damage resulting in reduced cardiac function and/or death) or CVA there can still be a beneficial protective effect. After a heart attack it has been shown that for the next 2–3 years there is a reduced risk of further MI and 20–25% reduction in all causes of death if patients had participated in an exercise rehabilitation programme.[4,22–25]
6. *Lifelong activity* is very important. Once regular activity ceases, for example after leaving school or college, *there is no protective effect later on in life*.[4,6] The benefits of physical activity cannot be 'put in the bank', but what can be 'saved' from a younger age is a positive attitude towards exercise and health.
7. *Exercise remains a vital intervention* in any treatment for CHD and CVA.
8. The *mode, frequency* and *duration* of exercise needs to be appropriate (prescribed) for the individual.[26,27]
9. *Exercise and physical activity have an independent protective effect*. Even without modifying risk factors such as alcohol, diet, obesity and

smoking, exercise on its own can reduce the likelihood of a person suffering an MI. This demonstrates that the adoption of regular exercise as an intervention has an *independent* effect in the protection against CHD and CVA.[13,16]

As sedentary living is a common risk factor for both CHD and CVA it seems sensible to suggest that these conditions will respond to the same type of physical activity strategy, and in fact this has been shown to be the case in the specific sections of this chapter.

The cost of CHD and CVA

It was stated previously that CHD and CVA are the major causes of premature death and disabling disease in the UK, Europe, USA and Canada, along with other developed countries.[1] In Figure 2.2, the proportions of CHD and CVA are compared with other fatal diseases.

In 1991, the estimated cost of Britain's Health Service for treating CHD was £917 million.[28] In addition to the various financial costs of CHD and CVA on society, it is also very important to acknowledge the less quantifiable costs – personal, emotional and social costs where family members or friends are also affected.

Beliefs and attitudes

To this point the discussion has focused on the health benefits of regular participation in physical activity and exercise. Research has now highlighted the impact of people's beliefs and attitudes towards physical activity. It has acknowledged the balance between individual perceptions, motivation and the possible impact of an evolving techno-mechanical society which allows individuals to live less actively, as further discussed in Chapter 7. If people's beliefs and attitudes towards health and exercise can clearly be identified, then possible strategies to increase widespread participation can be implemented.

In 1992, a major English study was published which highlighted people's beliefs and attitudes towards exercise, heart disease and stroke.[30] This study, *The Allied Dunbar National Fitness Survey* (ADNFS), investigated 6000 adults in England, aged 16–74 years. A six-point rating scale from 0 to 5 (0 being the lowest) was used to determine the amount and intensity of activity performed and the number of bouts of exercise in these categories undertaken in the previous 4 weeks. The results were:

- 80% of people surveyed believed that exercise was beneficial,
- 61% of men and 69% of women in activity level 0 *actually believed* themselves to be fit,
- 47% of men and 57% of women in activity level 0 *actually believed* themselves to be active,
- 70% of men and 91% of women were not active enough to gain a health benefit.

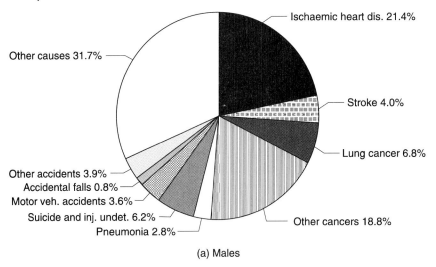

(a) Males

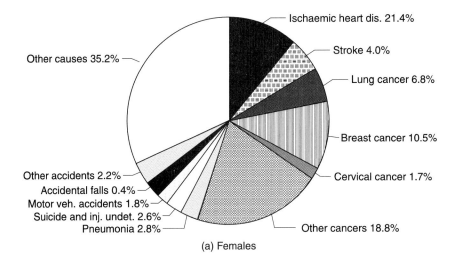

(a) Females

Figure 2.2 Cause of death up to age 75, England 1993–1994. (a) males; (b) females. (From PHCDS,[29] by courtesy of the National Institute of Epidemiology.)

This research highlights the low or non-existent levels of activity within a large representative group of the English population, in spite of their belief in the health benefits of exercise. It also indicates that these individuals did not have an understanding of the minimum level of exercise that is beneficial.

England's Health Education Authority's own publication *Health Gain News*[31] voiced concern over strategies advocated to improve activity participation levels across all society. It suggested that the most successful trials were those that incorporated home-based activities such as walking. When regular attendance to more structured exercise sessions were required there were more problems with compliance but, as will be discussed further in Chapters 3 and 7, when quality guidance and supervision are given, as an integral part of structured exercise, adherence rates significantly improve. If participation in activity and exercise is to be maintained and enjoyable, exercise professionals must be knowledgeable, flexible to people's participation constraints, creative and practical, in order to adapt advice to each individual client. If it is enjoyable and the benefits are made clear, a lifelong behaviour to activity is more likely to be adopted and sustained.

Fifty years of research concludes that regular physical activity has a protective effect against heart disease and stroke. With such benefits now so widely known and the resulting public health problem remaining vast, there is much to be done to swing not just social opinion but social behaviour into substantially increasing weekly amounts of physical activity in people's lives. As discussed further in Chapter 7, it appears that a similar approach to the very strong anti-smoking campaign may be required – one that confronts people on a regular basis. Some important underlining strategies for behavioural intervention to increase participation will be discussed in Chapter 3 and applying those changes in real situations in Chapter 7.

How much activity is enough to modify the risk factors?

In order to determine how much activity is required to modify the risk factors, standardized measurements must be applied. Such beneficial levels of exercise, as summarized in Chapter 1 (see Figure. 1.3) can be described in numerous ways and include:

- the number of calories expended per day,
- the time spent being active at a percentage of a person's aerobic capacity or at a MET equivalent (one MET represents the approximate rate of oxygen consumption of a seated adult),[32,33]
- the amount of light, moderate or vigorous activities performed,
- the amount of time spent being active at a specific rating of perceived exertion (RPE).

Further explanation of these physiological terms are found in Chapters 4–6.

Two key studies which illustrate a positive dose–response relationship between levels of activity and reduction in the incidence of CHD and CVA are the San Franciscan dockers study and the British Regional Heart Study.

The classic *San Franciscan longshoremen (dockers) study* of 3686 men compared those in heavy manual labour with those in work of a lower intensity. The higher manual labour men burned approximately 1000 more calories per day than those in low-intensity labour. This is equivalent to $1\frac{1}{2}$ hours of steady walking per day. The low-energy output men had an 80% increased risk of fatal heart attack compared with those in high-energy output jobs.[2,34]

The *British Regional Heart Study*[16] of 7735 middle-aged men looked at a variety of lifestyle behaviours. As part of this study, the men were categorized according to their activity levels, taking into account the type, intensity, frequency and duration of participation in physical activity. A physical activity index was developed depending on the subjects' participation levels. The categories were vigorous, moderately vigorous, moderate, light occasional, or inactive.

The main findings were that those men who reported high activity levels had reduced incidence of CHD and CVA. Even in those men who reported lower intensity but regular activity, such as gardening or pleasure walking, a reduced risk of heart attack was still demonstrated.

The justification for recommending low-intensity exercise, which may not necessarily lead to a discernible level of improved fitness, has been given a new perspective by the publication of the consensus opinion of a panel of experts in the field of physical activity and health.[33] The 'new' recommendation now considers health in relation to physical activity rather than just specific cardiorespiratory fitness. This is not to say, however, that the pursuit of improved cardiorespiratory fitness is by any means redundant within health promotion.

Discerning the difference: activity for health and exercise for fitness

In Chapter 1 the differences between daily physical activity and structured exercise were acknowledged. It is important that exercise and health professionals clearly understand that such documents like those set out by the American College of Sports Medicine's Position Stand – 'a recommendation for cardiorespiratory fitness' – are specifically for improving fitness,[26] but that health gains are also achieved alongside fitness improvements. More recent benchmark documents, including the 1996 *US Surgeon General's Report* and the *American Medical Association Report* by Pate *et al.*[33], set out the more minimal levels of activity in daily life which can confer a health benefit but not necessarily a noticeable fitness gain. Such health gains associated with lower levels of regular activity have included beneficial modifications to:

- blood lipids,
- hypertension,
- body composition,
- non-insulin-dependent diabetes mellitus (NIDDM),
- psychological function.

Contemporary recommendations

Guidelines for improved cardiorespiratory fitness, as also discussed in Chapter 4 onwards, are mainly concerned with reaching a level of intensity above 50% of an individual's aerobic capacity for a specified period at least 2–3 times per week. For health gain or improved risk factor profile for such conditions listed above, the more contemporary consensus focuses on the *total amount of energy expended on a daily basis with minimal bouts lasting 8–10 minutes accumulating to a total of 30 minutes per day most days of the week.* The specific mode and intensity of activity for improving health are not so important as when trying to improve fitness.[33] The 'new' recommendations help remove some of the perceived barriers to activity for those individuals with other physical (muscle/joint problems) or social constraints (lack of access to recreational facilities). The first part of Chapter 7 is specifically devoted to this topic.

Risk factor modification and exercise

The individual risk factors affected by physical activity (or lack of) which will be discussed include:

- blood lipids (fats and cholesterol),
- NIDDM,
- hypertension,
- obesity,
- cigarette smoking,
- fibrinogen.

Exercise and blood lipids

The word 'lipid' is derived from the Greek word *lipos*, meaning fat. Lipids come in various forms, including cholesterol and triglycerides, and problems arise if their level in the blood stream becomes too high.[12] Cholesterol is a necessary and vital constituent of cell walls, organelles and specialized tissue products and as such is very important for tissue function. In order for lipids (cholesterol and triglycerides) to be transported in the blood they need to be attached to protein, hence the term 'lipoprotein'. Cholesterol has more recently been divided into two main types, high-density lipoprotein cholesterol (HDL) and low-density lipoprotein cholesterol (LDL). Just looking at the levels of 'total cholesterol' present in the blood stream is now known not to be the key factor for determining CHD risk. In simple terms, high levels of LDL and low levels of HDL are 'bad', and lower levels of LDL and higher levels of HDL are 'good'.[12]

LDL-bound cholesterol

Low-density lipoproteins are part of the mechanism for transportation of cholesterol to the tissues. Raised levels of LDL can lead to an accumulation of lipids on artery walls, causing the development of atherosclerotic plaque. This plaque progressively narrows the artery and restricts the flow of blood. When this process occurs in the heart's coronary arteries there is a much heightened risk of a heart attack and blockage of blood to the heart muscle. *Angina* is the term used to describe chest pain associated with a narrowing of the blood flow through the coronary artery(ies), which has resulted from lipid-based atherosclerotic plaque.[11]

HDL-bound cholesterol

High-density lipoproteins are involved in reverse cholesterol transport, where they act as a vehicle for the removal of excess blood-borne lipids, taking them to the liver to be metabolized.[11,19,35]

A blood profile, therefore, that shows high total cholesterol (TC), and high LDL combined with low levels of HDL, is indicative of a high risk of developing atherosclerotic heart disease and subsequent MI (heart attack).[35,36] Another important factor is the ratio between HDL and LDL, which provides further insight into the likely risk of an individual developing heart disease.[20,35–38]

The effect of exercise on cholesterol

Higher levels of LDL (the so-called 'bad' cholesterol) are found in those who are sedentary and/or overweight.[36] By combining a low fat diet with regular exercise, a reduction in adverse blood lipoproteins has been shown.[36] Furthermore, there are the benefits of a reduction in the build-up of atherosclerotic plaque, an improvement in body mass index and an increase in exercise capacity, all of which have effects on other risk factors.[24,25,39,40] Higher levels of HDL have been found in those individuals who report levels of habitual physical activity of a moderate to vigorous nature. Further analysis of studies now allows health and exercise professionals to support the recommendation that daily low to moderate intensity exercise can also positively affect the HDL:LDL ratio.[9,17–20,33,35,41]

Types of activity and blood lipid profiles

It is important to recognize that certain types of activity or exercise training are more beneficial than others in improving blood lipid profiles. The majority of the research has established a beneficial link with aerobic-type activity and improved blood lipid profiles, but there is less evidence linking these benefits with high-resistance strength-training programmes.[42–44] Circuit-type exercise of low resistance and high repetitions of longer duration has, however, shown to have beneficial links with blood lipid profiles. Similar recommendations can be made in relation to hypertension, as will be discussed later in the chapter.

Above are some of the many studies that support the protective action of HDLs against CHD and the strong relationship that there is between regular aerobic activity and blood levels of HDL. Many of these studies also support the stance that habitual physical activity is one of the easiest and cheapest methods to achieve an improved lipid profile, namely raised blood HDL levels.[6,17]

Exercise and diabetes

Diabetes is a complex disorder and much research continues to further understand it. In simple terms it is a disorder which affects the regulation of blood sugar and the uptake of glucose (a carbohydrate) by the body's tissues. It is known that two main hormones produced in the pancreas, *insulin* and *glucagon*, are the key agents in controlling blood glucose. Insulin is required to facilitate the transport of glucose from the blood into the body's cells. Both types of diabetes, as described below, are due to deficiency or lack of effectiveness of insulin in transporting glucose into the body's cells.

The two forms of diabetes are:

1. *Type I, insulin-dependent diabetes mellitus (IDDM)*. This usually occurs during childhood. Type I diabetes occurs because the cells of the pancreas, where insulin is produced, are destroyed due to factors which are beyond the realms of this book. More important is the fact that, subsequently, individuals with IDDM, need to have daily insulin supplements for the rest of their lives.
2. *Type II, non-insulin-dependent diabetes mellitus (NIDDM)*. This is a condition which is usually 'acquired' in adults older than 40 years and is more prevalent in males.[45] It is strongly associated with a poor lifestyle in individuals who are inactive, overweight or obese.[21,46] Not only does NIDDM result in insufficient insulin production by the pancreas, but the body's cells develop a resistance to insulin which restricts the uptake of glucose. Other health conditions associated with NIDDM are hypertension and raised cholesterol,[21] which illustrates why it has links with the risk factors of CHD. NIDDM is thus a secondary risk factor for CHD,[11] of which predisposing factors include:

- obesity,
- increasing age,
- family history of diabetes.

The results from the *Health Survey for England* study,[45] which were then extrapolated to the whole of the UK, showed that between 1 035 000 and 1 242 000 people suffer from NIDDM. This equates to 3% of the population.[47] There is a similar prevalence in the USA, where approximately 10 million people have NIDDM.[11]

Physical activity, exercise and NIDDM

At rest, muscle cells like other cells in people with NIDDM are resistant to insulin, which prevents the uptake of glucose. During exercise, however, it has been shown that the activation of muscle contraction actually facilitates the uptake of glucose much like insulin, by making the muscle cells more permeable or allowing glucose to pass into the cells more easily.[48] The evidence at present suggests that it is during each individual bout of exercise that insulin resistance is lowered but, to date, longer term changes to insulin resistance have not been shown. Those with NIDDM should therefore be encouraged to be frequently active, as noted in the first half of Chapter 7, in order to help control their NIDDM.[21,46]

If an adequate activity level and dietary control is not maintained, individuals with NIDDM are at an increased risk of developing CHD, CVA, hypertension and peripheral vascular disease (PVD is where the circulation to the lower limbs is impaired). For a much fuller explanation on the complex process of blood sugar regulation, a physiology text should be consulted.[11] This positive effect of regular exercise on NIDDM is independent of whether other risk factors for this condition are present or not.[21]

Main research in NIDDM and exercise

The *Pennsylvania Alumni Health Study* of 5990 men[21] found that between the years of 1962 and 1976, 2020 men developed NIDDM. Those men who had higher reported leisure-time activity levels were less likely to develop NIDDM. For each increase in energy expenditure of 2000 kcal per week, there was a reduction in the incidence of NIDDM by 24%. This equates to a daily half-hour bout of vigorous activity such as jogging or tennis, or 1 hour per day of a more moderate activity such as walking. In those men who had the higher risk for developing NIDDM, exercise showed a greater protective effect in preventing its onset. In a large study with women, similar effects were noted.[46]

The *Second International Consensus Symposium on Physical Activity, Fitness and Health* stated that 'increased physical activity is associated with a reduced incidence of type II diabetes – NIDDM'.

It is considered that the adoption of regular physical activity may:

- prevent the onset of NIDDM in those at risk,
- reduce the medication requirement,
- reduce the risk of CHD when NIDDM has occurred.[49]

Exercise and hypertension

Hypertension (high blood pressure) is the major risk factor for CVA (stroke) and a primary risk factor for CHD. Because this book is about activity and cardiovascular health, a separate chapter (Chapter 6) discusses considerations of hypertension. In general, hypertension can be modified by exercise and is linked to the onset of NIDDM.[11,21] Its prevalence in Western societies affects about 20% of the adult population.[45,50,51] The prevalence of hypertension and its links to inactivity or the benefits to reducing hypertension have specifically been recognized by the American College of Sports Medicine in a specific opinion 'Position Stand'.[27]

Exercise and obesity

Obesity can be defined objectively when the ratio between body surface area and weight exceeds a certain level.[32] This ratio is known as the

Table 2.1 Standard figures for BMI. (From OPCS[52])

Descriptor	Index (BMI)
Underweight	20 or less
Average	>20–25
Overweight	>25–30
Obese	>30

body mass index (BMI), calculated by body weight (kg) divided by height squared (BMI = kg/m^2). BMI is highly correlated with body fat and gives a better estimate of body fat than weight alone.[11] Table 2.1 shows standard figures for BMI; the higher the figure the higher the risk of CHD/CVA.

BMI, body fat and body shape

As illustrated above, possession of a high BMI is a risk factor for CHD/CVA, but some caution must be taken in light of an individual's physique and exercise history. Knowing a person's percentage body fat helps clarify how the total body weight is made up. It is possible that someone who is a body-builder with very large and heavy muscles could have a high BMI, which is neither a function of adipose tissue (fat) nor a risk of developing CHD.

Obesity is a modifiable risk factor for CVD, and is strongly associated with NIDDM and hypertension. The problem is complex in that there are many factors that interact, both psychological and physiological, and so strategies that may be used to try to reduce body weight may not always be simple.[53] In the 1997 annual J.B. Woolfe Lecture of the American College of Sports Medicine, Professor Claude Bouchard summarized from various research that between 25% and 40% of obesity could be linked to genetic factors. Such a figure still leaves a large proportion of the remaining 60% to include behaviour (e.g. diet and activity).

The distribution of adipose tissue is predictive of CHD. It is interesting to note that an 'apple-shaped' or 'pot belly' distribution of fat in the abdominal region typically seen in men (which some females can also demonstrate) is strongly associated with CHD, whereas a 'pear-shaped' distribution more often seen in women, has less association. A more objective description of apple- or pear-shaped fat distribution is the use of the waist to hip girth ratio, where a ratio of greater than 1.0 in men and 0.8 in women is predictive of CHD.[54]

Research findings on obesity and exercise

In 1993 the Health Education Authority[55] published the figures below which show that in Britain the population trend is for increasing weight. This has implications for the incidence of CHD, CVA, hypertension and NIDDM, for which excess weight as a risk factor has already been discussed.

Aged 16–64
1980 males 30% overweight, 6% obese
      females 32% overweight, 8% obese
1992 males 48% overweight, 8% obese
      females 40% overweight, 13% obese

Niebauer et al.[39] took a group of 18 symptomatic CHD patients and studied them for 5 years. They were placed on a low-fat diet and participated in a prescribed aerobic exercise programme (30 minutes a day on a cycle ergometer at home, and 2–4 group sessions a week of 60 minutes). Compared with a control group, after 1 year the subject group showed a reduction in total cholesterol, LDL and triglycerides. After 5 years all CHD risk factors were much improved, including weight and BMI.

Two one-year trials involving high levels of activity, alone or in combination with dietary control have shown reductions in body fat and improvements in HDL.[36]

The Health Education Authority's *Health Update 5*[56] quotes several pieces of research that support physical activity as a method of improving weight reduction, some of which have shown benefit with less intense activity than the studies described above. For example, one study used brisk walking for 5 days a week plus dietary control and found this to be effective for a group of moderately obese women.[57]

From the studies described above it can be seen that alterations in diet that reduce calorific and fat intake, combined with increased energy expenditure, will decrease weight and body fat, but the level of motivation and support given must be extremely high for benefit to be seen and maintained. It must be recognized, as further described in Chapter 3, that the maintenance of weight loss by an individual often fails for many psychological and social reasons and the exercise professional can play a key role in the motivation and adherence of a client to an exercise and diet regime.[57]

Exercise and cigarette smoking

Attitudes toward smoking and exercise

The *Health Education Monitoring Survey 1995*[58] looked at the knowledge, attitudes and behaviour of adults (aged 16–74 years, in England) towards a variety of health-related behaviours. These included smoking and physical activity. In relation to smoking:

- 84% knew that smoking was a risk factor for CHD,
- 55% knew that it was a risk factor for stroke,
- 68% would like to give up smoking,
- 35% said that they intended to give up within the next year.

The *Health of the Nation* White Paper[59] stated that cigarette smoking is the main risk factor for CHD, stroke and PVD. Combining these diseases together with adverse lipid profiles, high dietary intake of saturated fats and hypertension accounted for up to 18% of deaths from CHD and 11% of deaths from stroke.

One possible way that cigarette smoking can negatively affect our vascular system is via the effect on fibrinogen, a blood clotting factor. Nicotine and carbon monoxide from cigarette smoke have been identified as the main products that negatively affect the cardiovascular system. Cigarette smoking reduces HDL cholesterol and increases fibrinogen levels. When fibrinogen levels are raised too high, the blood becomes more viscous (sticky) and acts much like a scaffolding on which lipids can accumulate and cause arterial narrowing due to atheroma formation.[60]

It is obvious that exercise professionals are in a position to participate in smoking cessation programmes, but should ensure that this is backed by recognized counselling training. A possible approach is for exercise professionals to collaborate with clinicians who lead smoking cessation and health promotion programmes.

Because exercise professionals may see clients/patients on a more regular basis, they are in an excellent position to provide more frequent encouragement and support to those attempting to give up or who have recently stopped smoking.

The link between exercise, healthier lifestyles and smoking

At this point there are two important questions that arise: Is there a relationship between a healthy lifestyle and a reduced likelihood of smoking? Would fewer individuals smoke if they were more physically active?

There is evidence, from large population studies, that those individuals with higher physical activity levels are more likely to lead a healthier lifestyle which also includes a healthy diet and the avoidance of smoking. The *British Regional Heart Study* again found some key findings in addition to the effects of physical activity on lowering the incidence of CHD. It found that the more inactive men tended to be smokers.[16]

A large study of 2907 adults done in the Netherlands[8] found that their 'fit' subjects were less likely to smoke. Lower body fat and less smoking were significantly related to those men and women who participated in sports activity.

Continuing analyses of 14786 Harvard Graduates in the USA[4] show that in relation to smoking habits, participation in an active lifestyle and stopping cigarette smoking gave a longer lifespan. This conclusion was based on data from non-smokers, who were physically active and from those who had given up the smoking habit and had begun regular physical activity.

As previously stated, it has been found that on cessation of smoking there is a progressive reduction in risk for CHD in 2–3 years.[14] It must be appreciated, however, that the relationship between physical activity and smoking is not a simple one, and that suitable interventions to promote cessation should continue to be advocated.[61]

Exercise and fibrinogen

As stated in the earlier section on smoking, raised fibrinogen levels can be considered a major cardiovascular health risk. Douglas *et al.*[62] reviewed the effects of exercise on atherosclerotic heart disease in women and highlighted the links between smoking, fibrinogen levels, platelet aggregation and other clotting factors. Elevated fibrinogen levels have been associated with inactivity in combination with other clotting mechanisms.[63,64] Kannel *et al.*,[65] in the ongoing Framingham studies, with 1315 subjects, found that raised fibrinogen levels were more strongly associated with CHD and stroke in men than women, but women were still negatively affected.

Cross-sectional studies and longitudinal studies strongly suggest that exercise reduces plasma fibrinogen levels by 0.4 g/l over several months.[66] In addition to fibrinogen, lower levels of body fat and triglyceride lipids were associated with greater aerobic fitness and total daily energy expenditure; thus showing a positive relationship between fibrinogen, other risk factors for CHD and exercise.[9]

Research over decades has provided us with the knowledge that one of the most simple and effective interventions to combat heart disease and stroke is to be regularly active. To date, there still lies ahead the challenge of persuading the majority of the population of industrialized nations to alter their lifestyles sufficiently to prevent premature sickness and death related to CHD and CVA.

References

1. World Health Organisation (1991) World Health Statistics Annual. In *Health Update 1*, Health Education Authority, 1993.
2. Paffenbarger, R.S., Laughlin, M.E., Gima, A.S. *et al.* (1970) Work activity of longshoremen as related to death from coronary heart disease and stroke. *New Engl. J. Med.*, **282**, 1109–1114.
3. Paffenbarger, R.S., Hyde, R.T., Wing, A.L. and Hsieh, C. (1986) Physical activity, all-cause mortality, and longevity of college alumni. *New Engl. J. Med.*, **314**, 605–613.
4. Paffenbarger, R.S., Kampert, J.B. and Lee, I-Min. (1994) Changes in physical activity and other lifeway patterns influencing longevity. *Med. Sci. Sports Exerc.*, **26**, 857–865.
5. Morris, J.N., Heady, J.A. and Raffle, P.A.B. (1953) Coronary heart disease and the physical activity of work. *Lancet*, **ii**, 1053–1057, 1111–1120.
6. Morris, J.N. (1994) Exercise in the prevention of coronary heart disease: today's best buy in public health. *Med. Sci. Sports Exerc.*, **26**, 807–814.
7. Powell, K.E. and Blair, S.N. (1994) The public health burdens of sedentary living habits: theoretical but realistic estimates. *Med. Sci. Sports Exerc.*, **26**, 851–856.

8. Bovens, A.M., Van Baak, M., Vrenken, J.G. *et al.* (1993) Physical activity, fitness, and selected risk factors for CHD in active men and women. *Med. Sci. Sports Exerc.*, **25**, 572–576.

9. Rauramaa, R., Tuomainen, P., Vaisanen, S. and Rankinen, T. (1995) Physical activity and health-related fitness in middle-aged men. *Med. Sci. Sports Exerc.*, **27**, 707–712.

10. Lakka, T.A., Venalainen, J.M., Rauramaa, R. *et al* (1994) Relation of leisure-time physical activity and cardiorespiratory fitness to the risk of acute myocardial infarction in men. *New Engl. J. Med.*, **330**, 1549–1554.

11. Wilmore, J.H. and Costill, D.L. (1994) *Physiology of Sport and Exercise*, Human Kinetics, Champaign, IL.

12. Pollock, M.L. and Schmidt, D.H. (eds) (1995) *Heart Disease and Rehabilitation*, Human Kinetics, Champaign, IL.

13. Paffenbarger, R.S., Wing, A.L. and Hyde, R.T. (1978). Physical activity as an index of heart attack risk in college alumni. *Am. J. Epidemiol.*, **108**, 161–175.

14. Rosenberg, L., Palmer, J.R. and Shapiro, S. (1990) Decline in the risk of myocardial infarction among women who have stopped smoking. *New Engl. J. Med.*, **322**, 213–217.

15. Wannemethee, G. and Shaper, A.G. (1992) Physical activity and stroke in British middle-aged men. *Br. Med. J.*, **304**, 597–601.

16. Shaper, A.G. and Wannamethee, G. (1991) Physical activity and ischaemic heart disease in middle-aged British men. *Br. Heart J.*, **66**, 384–394.

17. Davison, R.C. and Grant, S. (1993) Is walking sufficient exercise for health? *Sports Med.*, **16**, 369–373.

18. Pay, R. C, Hardman, A.E., Jones, G.J.W. and Hudson, A. (1992) The acute effects of low-intensity exercise on plasma lipids in endurance-trained and untrained young adults. *Eur. J. Appl. Physiol.*, **64**, 182–186.

19. Higuchi, M., Tamai, T. and Ohta, T. (1994) Effects of exercise on plasma lipid metabolism and exercise therapy of hyperlipidaemia. *Med. Exerc. Nutr. Health*, **3**, 308–316.

20. Dannenberg, A.L., Keller, J.B. and Wilson, P.W.F. (1989) Leisure time physical activity in the Framingham offspring study: description, seasonal variation, and risk factor correlates. *Am. J. Epidemiol.*, **129**, 76–88.

21. Helmrich, S.P., Ragland, D.R. and Paffenbarger, R.S. (1994) Prevention of non-insulin-dependent diabetes mellitus with physical activity. *Med. Sci. Sports Exerc.*, **26**, 824–830.

22. O'Connor, G.T., Buring, J.E. and Yusuf, S. *et al.* (1989) An overview of randomised trials of rehabilitation with exercise after myocardial infarction. *Circulation*, **80**, 234–244.

23. Oldridge, N.B., Guyatt, G.H., Fischer, M.E. and Rimm, A.A. (1988) Cardiac rehabilitation after myocardial infarction: combined experience of randomised clinical trials. *J. Am. Med. Assoc.*, **260**, 945–950.

24. Hambrecht, R., Niebauer, J., Marburger, C. *et al.* (1993) Various intensities of leisure time physical activity in patients with coronary artery disease: effects on cardiorespiratory fitness and progression of coronary atherosclerotic lesions. *J. Am. Coll. Cardiol.*, **22**(2), 468–477.

25. Quinn, T.G., Alderman, E.L., McMillan, A. and Haskell, W. (1994) Development of new coronary atherosclerotic lesions during a 4 year multifactor risk reduction program: the Stanford coronary risk intervention project (SCRIP). *J. Am. Coll. Cardiol.*, **24**, 900–908.

26. American College of Sports Medicine (1990) Position Stand: The recommended quantity and quality of exercise for developing and maintaining

cardiorespiratory and muscular fitness in healthy adults. *Med. Sci. Sports Exerc.*, **22**(2), 265–274.

27. American College of Sports Medicine (1993) Position Stand: physical activity, physical fitness, and hypertension. *Med. Sci. Sports Exerc.*, **25**, i–x.
28. Office of Health Economics (1992) In *Health Update 1*, 1993 Health Education Authority.
29. Public Health Common Data Set for England (1995) Produced by National Institute of Epidemiology (formerly the Institute of Public Health), University of Surrey.
30. Health Education Authority, Sports Council (1992) *Allied Dunbar National Fitness Survey*.
31. Health Education Authority (1996) *Health Gain News*, no. 3, 1.
32. Ainsworth, B.E., Haskell, W.L., Leon, A.S. *et al.* (1993) Compendium of physical activities: classification of energy costs of human physical activities. *Med. Sci. Sports Exerc.*, **25**, 71–80.
33. Pate, R.R., Pratt, M., Blair, S.N. *et al.* (1995) Physical activity and public health. A recommendation from the Centres for Disease Control and Prevention and the American College of Sports Medicine. *J. Am. Med. Assoc.*, **273**, 402–407.
34. Paffenbarger, R.S. and Hale, W.E. (1975) Work activity and coronary heart mortality. *New Engl. J. Med.*, **292**, 545–550.
35. Campaigne, B., Fontaine, R.N. and Park, Y.C. (1993) Reverse cholesterol transport with acute exercise. *Med. Sci. Sports Exerc.*, **25**, 1346–1351.
36. Wood, P.D. (1994) Physical activity, diet and health: independent and interactive effects. *Med. Sci. Sports Exerc.*, **26**, 838–843.
37. Morris, J.N., Kagen, A., Pattison, D.C. *et al.* (1966) Incidence and prediction of ischaemic heart disease in London busmen. *Lancet*, **2**(463), 553–559.
38. Lakka, T.A., Venalainen, J.M., Rauramaa, R. *et al.* (1994) Relation of leisure-time physical activity and cardiorespiratory fitness to the risk of acute myocardial infarction in men. *New Engl. J. Med.*, **330**, 1549–1554.
39. Niebauer, J., Hambrecht, R., Schlierf, G. *et al.* (1994) Five years of physical exercise and low fat diet: effects on progression of coronary artery disease. *J. Cardiopul. Rehab.*, **15**, 47–64.
40. Haskell, W.L., Alderman, E.L., Fair, J.M. *et al.* (1994) Effects of multiple risk factor reduction on coronary atherosclerosis and clinical cardiac events in men and women with coronary artery disease. *Circulation*, **89**, 975–990.
41. Eaton, C.B., Lapane, K.L., Garber, C.E. *et al.* (1995) Physical activity, physical fitness, and coronary heart disease risk factors. *Med. Sci. Sports Exerc.*, **27**, 340–346.
42. Wallace, M.B., Moffat, R.J., Haymes, E.M. and Green, N.R. (1991) Acute effects of resistance exercise on parameters of lipoprotein metabolism. *Med. Sci. Sports Exerc.*, **23**, 199–204.
43. Kohl, H.W., Gordon, N.F. and Scott, C.B., (1992) Musculoskeletal strength and serum lipid levels in men and women. *Med. Sci. Sports. Exerc.*, **24**, 1080–1087.
44. Kokkinos, P.F., Hurley, B.F., Smutok, M.A. *et al.* (1991) Strength training does not improve lipid profiles in men at risk for coronary heart disease. *Med. Sci. Sports Exerc.*, **23**, 1134–1139.
45. Bennet, N. (1993) *Health Survey for England*, Department of Health, London.

46. Manson, J.E., Rimm, E.B. and Stampfer, M.J. (1991) Physical activity and incidence of non-insulin dependent diabetes mellitus in women. *Lancet*, **338**, 774–778.
47. British Diabetic Association (1995) *Diabetes in the United Kingdom*, London.
48. Ivy, J.L. (1987) The insulin-like effect of muscle contraction. *Exerc. Sports Sci. Rev.*, **15**, 29–51.
49. Bouchard, C., Shepherd, R.J. and Stephens, T. (eds) (1992) *Consensus Statement*, Second International Consensus Symposium on Physical Activity, Fitness and Health. Human Kinetics, Champaign, IL.
50. Office of Population Census and Surveys (1992) *Health Update 5*, OPCS, London.
51. Lund-Johansen, P. (1982) Physical activity and hypertension. *Scand. J. Soc. Med.*, **S29**, 185–194.
52. Office of Population Census and Surveys (1990) *Health Update 1*, OPCS, London.
53. Miller, W. (1991) Obesity: diet composition energy expenditure, and treatment of the obese patient. *Med. Sci. Sports Exerc.*, **23**, 273–274.
54. Lapidus, L., Bengtsson, C., Larsson, B. *et al.* (1984) Distribution of adipose tissue and risk of cardiovascular disease in adults: a 12 year follow up of participants in the population study of women in Gothenburg, Sweden. *Br. Med. J.*, **289**, 1257–1261.
55. Health Education Authority (1993) Coronary heart disease. In *Health Update 1*, HEA, London.
56. Health Education Authority (1995) Physical activity. In *Health Update 5*, HEA, London.
57. Foreyt, J.P. and Goodrich, G.K. (1991) Factors common to successful therapy for the obese patient. *Med. Sci. Sports Exerc.*, **23**, 292–297.
58. Health Education Authority (1995) *Health Education Monitoring Survey*, Social Survey Division of the Office of Population Census and Surveys, London.
59. HMSO (1990) *Health of the Nation* (White Paper), HMSO, London.
60. Kannel, W.B., McGee, D.E.L. and Castelli, W.P. (1984) Latest perspective on cigarette smoking and cardiovascular disease: the Framingham study. *J. Cardiac Rehab.*, **4**, 267–277.
61. King, A.C., Blair, S.A.N., Bild, D.E. *et al.* (1992) Determinants of physical activity and interventions in adults. *Med. Sci. Sports Exerc.*, **26**, S223–S233.
62. Douglas, P., Clarkson, T.B. and Flowers, N.C. (1992) Exercise and atherosclerotic heart disease in women. *Med. Sci. Sports Exerc.*, **24**, S267–276.
63. Van Den Berg, P.J.M., Hospers, J.E.H., Van Liet, M. *et al.* (1997) Effect of endurance training and seasonal fluctuation on coagulation and fibrinolysis in young sedentary men. *J. Appl. Physiol.*, **82**(2), 613–620.
64. Eliasson, M., Asplund, K. and Evrin, P-E. (1996) Regular leisure time physical activity predicts high activity of tissue plasminogen activator: The Northern Sweden MONICA Study. *Int. J. Epidem.*, **25**, 1182–1188.
65. Kannel, W.B., Wolf, P.A., Castelli, W.P. and D'Agostino, R.B. (1987) Fibrinogen and risk of cardiovascular disease. The Framingham study. *J. Am. Med. Assoc.*, **258**, 9.
66. Ernst, E. (1993) Regular exercise reduces fibrinogen levels: a review of longitudinal studies. *Br. J. Sports Med.*, **27**, 175–176.

3
Psychological aspects of physical activity and exercise

*Part I Introduction to psychology and links with physical activity and
    exercise*
Psychology, physical activity and exercise
Part II Exercise, physical activity and mental well-being
The cost and benefits
Negative psychological aspects of physical activity and exercise
How physical activity may improve mental health – the mechanisms
Part III Developing the 'exercise habit'
Adherence to exercise
Behaviour–cues and consequences
Barriers to exercise and physical activity participation
Beliefs and attitudes about physical activity and exercise
The process of changing exercise behaviour
Chapter summary
References

There are three parts to this chapter, which aim to give a foundation of the links between psychology, mental well-being and factors affecting participation:

- Part I is an *introduction* to the subject of psychology and its links with physical activity and exercise.
- Part II covers the rudimentary elements of *mental well-being*, how mental well-being is affected by participating in physical activity and exercise. The concepts in this section provide a foundation for many of the concepts in Part III.
- Part III covers those psychological factors which influence or distract a person from *participating in activity*, through effective counselling interventions and dispelling misconceptions about activity, exercise and fitness.

Part I   Introduction to psychology and links with physical activity and exercise

There are many factors which may influence an individual's desire or ability to be more physically active. Psychology is a key influencing factor of life, alongside social, political, economic and biological aspects. As part of this complex structure of life, psychology has an important part to play. Psychology or 'the science of the human mind'[1] affects us in many ways, such as through our relationships with others and through the influences of local cultures and the laws and policies of the nation. Our psychological and social (psychosocial) health, responses and reactions to news and situations may be shaped by our beliefs and understandings, and the way we raise our children will be shaped by the way we were raised. Psychology has been involved from our earliest days as children, when beliefs and understandings of physical activity were first introduced and formed and how we responded to our natural physical abilities or inabilities.

Psychology is not a new science. Its roots can be traced back to several centuries BC when the great Greek philosophers posed such questions as: Do people perceive reality correctly? Are people capable of free choice? It was at about the same point in history that the 'father of medicine', Hippocrates, was making observations of how the brain controlled the functions of the body. These questions are equally valid now, and throughout this chapter the individual's perceptions and beliefs about the choices they have available to them with regard to being more physically active are discussed. What we would recognize today as 'psychology' began in the nineteenth century, when it was realized that the mind and behaviour could be studied scientifically. Thus, psychology may be more specifically defined as 'the scientific study of behaviour and mental processes'.[2] Exercise behaviour is one area that has begun to receive extensive research interest as a result of the benefits of physical activity being recognized. There are now five major approaches to the study of psychology:

- *Behavioural* – the behaviour itself is central, rather than the brain and nervous system.
- *Cognitive* – mental processes are studied to interpret behaviours.
- *Biological* – behaviour is related to electrical and chemical events inside the body.
- *Psychoanalytical* – behaviour stems from unconscious processes (such as beliefs, fears and desires).
- *Phenomenological* – description of the 'subjective experience'. Actions are in the control of the individual and not controlled by processed information or external forces. Motivation for personal 'growth'.

Each of these approaches does not necessarily exclude any of the others and each aspect may be recognized in this chapter. For example, a combination approach of cognitive and behavioural psychology may be applied to help a client become more active.

Psychology, physical activity and exercise

As the theme of this text is about effectively guiding individuals in activity for cardiovascular health, various psychological models and theories will be covered, looking mainly at aerobic-type activity.

For more extensive and in-depth discussion of the models, theories and research of exercise psychology, we would further recommend specialized exercise related psychology texts.[3-5]

The purpose of this chapter is to raise awareness of some of the many factors involved in the prescription of cardiovascular exercise and physical activity, and how some knowledge of these factors will help to guide interventions, and the type of exercise/physical activity programme that an exercise professional may design. The following paragraphs introduce some of these points.

Prescription of exercise and physical activity

From the discussions in various chapters it is evident that the delivery of exercise programmes should be specific and individualized to each client. That is, a programme must be capable of delivering what it sets out to achieve, and the person it is designed for must want and be able to comply with its requirements.

To ensure this, the exercise professional must be aware of what they are ultimately attempting to deliver for the client. Being 'on' an exercise programme may imply that at some point in the future it will cease, much like being on a diet. Failure is often the natural end-point. The consultation process (Chapter 12) provides an excellent means for the exercise professional to gauge the client's perception of the need for exercise to be a short, medium or long-term change. It is very important that physical activity and exercise are not perceived as a short-term 'fix', because as soon as the client becomes inactive, the benefits gained begin to disappear.

Ensuring that prescription has a positive connotation

The term 'exercise prescription', as with GP referral schemes in Britain, potentially carries negative connotations of being a temporary fix associated with illness, much like the prescription of a medication. A good consultation process includes the acknowledgement that the aims of activity are to prevent a reversal in health status and that the prescription is to act as a catalyst for achieving a positive result. Exercise and physical activity may not only be part of a 'cure', but also the means for long-term prevention. The exercise professional, therefore, has the responsibility to promote the benefits of being 'active for life', coupled with more immediate fitness gains and reduced state of illness. It should be expected that a client may wish to change the type and venue of exercise in time. An example from the authors' experience is of a man who attended an exercise centre over a period of 12 months. As he became confident that he could control his own activity, he decided to join the local hill-walking group, which for so long he had perceived to be beyond his abilities. To date, he continues his regular activity through hill-walking and is no longer attending the exercise centre.

The purpose of this example is to illustrate that although a health club may consider losing a client member to be a loss of business, the exercise professional should feel a sense of achievement by helping someone become more active and healthier. Such a situation represents a positive achievement, but all too often the exercise industry rates its success on 'membership retention' rather than client health and fitness achievements. It is very likely, however, that the client above will recommend others to the exercise professional and possibly a string of future clients will follow, which in the long run is likely to be more successful in financial business terms.

The evidence described in Chapter 2 makes it clear that being physically active is a requirement for reducing the risk of disease and that gains in fitness may only be temporary if the individual ceases 'doing fitness' at the required levels. Exercise programming should be designed to enable longer term adherence. This will incorporate an understanding of why a client may wish to become more active, e.g. to feel fitter, to lose weight, to socialize, or to enjoy, and why they may also feel that they are unable to become more active, e.g. no time, too fat, no facilities or does not have the 'correct' clothes.

The exercise professional must ensure that the client clearly understands that there is no form of 'bank' where fitness can be saved for a rainy day, but that even short duration bouts of physical activity and exercise, if carried out regularly and adhered to, can have a beneficial effect on long-term health.[6]

It is common for exercise professionals to speak of the benefits of exercise and physical activity in physical or physiological terms, such as changes in body composition or aerobic fitness. If, however, a client is asked to relate the benefits they have derived from exercise, particularly in the early stages of a programme, they are likely to explain changes from a psychological rather than a physical perspective by making such remarks as 'I *feel* better', 'I *feel* I have more energy', 'I *feel* less stressed'. Further on into their programme they may well offer descriptions of benefits in physical terms, such as of how they have lost weight, feel toned, and do not get as out of breath walking the dog or walking up hills. The reasons for the physical changes are described in Chapter 4 and how to set levels for both health and physical fitness improvement in Chapters 7 and 9. A client's perception of what they have achieved may change with time and shift from psychological remarks to a physiological focus, as that is what provides them with further reinforcement to continue to exhibit the pattern of behaviour.

Psychological importance in the first few weeks of becoming noticeably more active

Even after the initial consultation session or the first session of exercise, the exercise professional may receive very positive feedback from the client. There may be many reasons for this – the social interaction, the feeling that they have taken control of part of their life or simply because being involved in an organized programme is a step towards improving themselves.

Although there will obviously be no measurable physiological changes in these very early stages, the psychological impact that can be experienced by the exerciser can provide the exercise professional with an immediately useful 'tool' to aid the journey towards a positive and permanent change in behaviour, particularly over the first few weeks of the programme.

A main problem with the prescription of exercise is that people tend not to adhere to a programme for an extended period of time. With a commonly reported dropout rate of 50% within the first 6 months of the programme[3] it would seem that in order to encourage adherence, at least in the initial stages, it may be that the physiological targets require less emphasis and the psychological benefits be emphasized even more, as they are immediately available to the individual.

The exercise professional may be instrumental in helping the patient with this process, but there are other influences that may provide real or perceived barriers to participation in exercise. These factors will be discussed later in this chapter and outlined in Table 3.1.

It is probable that a practising exercise professional uses elements of psychology on a daily basis without even realizing it, perhaps by telling an exerciser that they have improved or structuring the programme so that it is enjoyable.

Comments from the client, such as 'I feel better', are likely to be the result of several factors, all of which may impact on mental well-being.

Part II Exercise, physical activity and mental well-being

The cost and benefits

Twenty per cent of the UK population suffer from serious affective or mood disorder at some time in their life.[7] With the cost of treating mental disorders such as depression and anxiety estimated at up to 20% of the total NHS expenditure, or £4 billion per annum,[8] an inexpensive alternative to conventional therapy may provide a useful contribution. Exercise and physical activity are time and cost effective compared with drug treatments, and may act as a preventative against future occurrences of mental health problems.[9]

The overwhelming bulk of research on exercise and mental health shows that there is a beneficial link, whether or not there is a clinical condition[10,11], and 90% of all studies support the use of exercise as an aid for combating depression and anxiety.[12] It seems possible that exercise can be used alone, or in conjunction with other therapies,[13] in the prevention and treatment of mental health conditions.

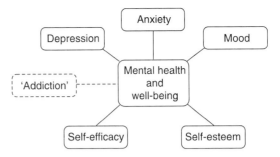

Figure 3.1 Aspects of mental health and well-being.

Several mental health benefits of exercise and physical activity have been found and the association is well established.[14] These include reductions in depression[15] and anxiety[16], as well as improved mood states,[17] increased self-esteem (self-concept)[18] and self-efficacy[19,20] (Figure 3.1). Each of these possible psychological aspects of exercise and physical activity will briefly be discussed.

Depression

Depression is a term used for a variety of states and is divided into two types. It can be a primary psychological disorder or secondary, such as when associated with eating disorders such as bulimia nervosa.[13] Both aerobic and non-aerobic (i.e. weight training) activities have been associated with reduced depression.[21,22] It has been found that aerobic activity may reduce depression more than a mixed or non-aerobic activity;[23] this is interesting to note, as many of the physiological benefits discussed in Chapter 4 are also derived from aerobic activity. This supports the notion of aerobic activity being a fundamental element of general exercise programmes for both physical and mental health.

Increased 'fitness' levels may enhance the antidepressant effect and a threshold of 15% improvement in cardiovascular fitness has been suggested before significant changes occur.[24] Reductions in levels of depression have also been found without any increase in fitness,[25] lending support to the potential effectiveness of low-intensity activity, where the effect is merely from participation, as discussed in Chapters 1, 2 and 7.

In an attempt to bring together the results of studies on the effect of exercise and depression, North and co-workers[13] looked at all the available research. Some of the main findings of their study were:

- long- and short-term exercise is effective at reducing depression – the effect may remain for some time,
- clinically and non-clinically depressed groups experience decreased depression with exercise,
- state (situation specific) and trait (general predisposition) depression decreases with exercise,
- all modes of exercise are effective,

- the longer the term of exercise, the longer the reduction in depression remains,
- exercise is as good or better than all known treatments.

It is possible that depression results from the repeated perception of having no control over the experiences of one's life. If a sense of control through being more active can be gained, the 'learned helplessness'[26] may be replaced by a 'sense of mastery'.[27] The exercise situation can promote the positive experiences necessary for this to occur if the programme has realistic preset goals which allow the client to gain a sense of achievement. It is evident that although physical activity and short-term exercise may have an antidepressant effect, for this effect to be longer term the exercise must be continued.

Anxiety

Anxiety is typically described in two ways: *trait anxiety* (a person's general 'day-to-day' predisposition towards anxiety), and *state anxiety* (the anxiety felt at a particular time in a particular situation – the level of trait anxiety may mediate this). The potential of aerobic exercise to reduce levels of state and trait anxiety has been widely researched and has been shown to be beneficial.[28,29]

Exercise of all types is as effective as traditional treatments for anxiety, although aerobic exercise is more beneficial than non-aerobic.[16] Reductions in levels of anxiety are available, without any measurable change in fitness, from a programme of exercise.[30]

Bouts of more than 20 minutes may be required to gain a significant reduction in the level of state anxiety. For a reduction in a person's trait anxiety to occur, the exercise must take place over at least 10 weeks and for best results 16 weeks. Larger anxiety-reducing effects have been shown for periods of exercise duration up to 30 minutes, although all periods of exercise have a positive effect,[16] including bouts as brief as 10 minutes.[31]

For the purposes of prescribing exercise for stress and anxiety reduction, the implications of these findings are that some exercise will be of benefit, but that a programme of aerobic exercise of 20–30 minutes' duration over a 10–16 week period is most likely to be of longer term benefit.

Moods

There is a clear link between exercise, positive mood and psychological well-being.[32] Even a single bout of exercise can enhance general mood[33] and positive mood changes are possible from different types of exercise.[34] However, while lower intensity exercise enhances positive mood,[35] high-intensity exercise has been found to reduce the level of positive mood state.[36] If a client perceives the amount or the intensity of the exercise to be too demanding, improvements in positive mood and psychological well-being may not occur.[37] Setting the appropriate intensity level is addressed in Chapters 7 and 9 (see also Chapter 6 for perceived exertion).

Low to moderate intensity programmes may then help to produce a more positive mood state which can aid longer term adherence to an exercise programme. This may be useful in the early stages of an exercise programme.

Improvements in fitness are not necessary for improving mood.[35] Therefore, emphasizing the performance of physical activity rather than the products of 'doing fitness', such as losing weight, can lead to a sense of mastery and increased self-esteem which could be reflected in better mental health and mood.

As different types of exercise have been associated with improved mood,[22,34,38] helping the client to choose an activity which they find enjoyable may encourage longer term adherence to the exercise.[39]

Self-esteem

Self-esteem is often regarded as the single most important measure of psychological well-being.[32] It may be defined as 'the awareness of good (excellence, goods) possessed by oneself',[40] or the feeling that you are an 'OK person', depending on your own definition of what 'good' and 'OK' are. Where self-concept is the picture a person builds up of their own identity, such as 'I am a man/woman', 'I am a provider', self-esteem is the individual's judgement of their own worth.[41] It has been experienced by the authors that an event such as a heart attack or serious accident which abruptly halts a person in carrying out their day-to-day responsibilities, can lead to a large reduction in their self-esteem. Exercise rehabilitation programmes are often used as a vehicle to help people regain self-esteem after such a physical and psychological blow.

Increases in levels of self-esteem have been found in different types of exercise,[18] although aerobic activity has been shown to be more beneficial.[42] Participating in physical activity and exercise can have a positive effect on these self-perceptions[43] and significant increases in self-esteem are related to participation in exercise[44] regardless of any other changes. This supports the importance of pursuing regular participation as the first goal for the client, by the prescription of appropriate levels of cardiovascular exercise for each individual.

The mechanism for the changes in self-esteem may be the gaining of a 'sense of mastery' and the perception of positive changes in fitness levels or psychological well-being. Various aspects of self-esteem pertaining to exercise have been identified in a hierarchical form with overall ('global') self-esteem as the top level encompassing all areas of life.[45] The next level is based on physical self-worth and is supported by several specific aspects of self-esteem known as 'subdomains'.

These subdomains include sports competence, body attractiveness, physical strength and physical condition. Each individual has their own perception of each of these aspects of themselves and having a high level of self-esteem in one domain does not necessarily mean that a client will have a similar level of self-esteem in other domains. For example, a client may have a high level of self-esteem about their physical condition, but not about how attractive their body is.

Based on this example, it should be noted that if an individual does not perceive it as important to be attractive, then it is unlikely that they will feel a reduced level of self-esteem as a result of this. If, however, a person feels that having an attractive body is very important, then their self-esteem will be affected if this condition is not what they would wish. The same principle applies for all of the subdomains.

A client's specific perception of themselves can be identified and influenced through behavioural interventions as part of the exercise programme.[46] The exercise professional may also be able to help the client find those activities which deliver the greatest returns in self-esteem as a means to promoting more prolonged adherence.

Self-efficacy/self-confidence

Self-efficacy is a person's 'judgement of their capabilities to organize and execute courses of action required to attain designated types of performances'.[20] It is a form of *self-confidence* which is specific to a particular situation, such as exercise. As self-confidence is a global belief that you will be successful in all situations, a person may be generally self-confident, but have a low level of self-efficacy (confidence) for exercise situations.

Self-efficacy theory[19] proposes that self-efficacy, the belief or expectation that the exercise may be successfully performed, is the mediator of all changes in exercise behaviour. As will be discussed later, the confidence to resist temptation to deviate from the desired behaviour is also important.

Self-efficacy, however, is generally considered to be a relatively poor predictor of exercise activity, adherence and dropout, and should be viewed alongside other theories when predictions of exercise activity are made.

The confidence to be able to participate in exercise is based on past learning and the individual's perceptions of what is required or expected from their exercise programme.

Figure 3.2 demonstrates how self-efficacy theory is based on two types of expectation:

- efficacy expectations – the beliefs that the behaviour can be performed,
- outcome expectations – beliefs about the 'product' of following the behaviour.

From the illustration it can be seen that a person is linked to the exercise behaviour by their beliefs that they can perform the desired tasks, such as participation on a regular basis. The behaviour must then precede the outcome that the client expects to occur, such as reducing weight (fat). This theory emphasizes how it is necessary to develop the process of behaviour by encouraging expectations based on the performance of the behaviour.

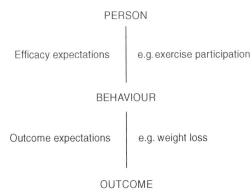

Figure 3.2 Expectations and outcomes related to exercise. (Adapted from Bandura, in Biddle and Mutrie[5] with permission.)

An example of this would be to encourage a client to consider three episodes of activity in a week to be a success, rather that look to what they ultimately may want to gain, i.e. weight loss. Weight (fat) loss may take some time to achieve and may be adversely affected by factors other than exercise, such as eating excessively.

If the client focuses on the weight loss initially, they may perceive an element of failure if the weight is not lost immediately. By focusing on the participation, three sessions in a week will be perceived as a success and a repeat of the behaviour is more likely. Ultimately the outcome expectations may be attained.

In order to reach the point of a product or outcome, such as the weight loss shown in Figure 3.2, the (efficacy) expectation that they are capable of participation in exercise must first be achieved as the basis for the development of the exercise behaviour. If a client does not have the confidence to begin or continue to exercise, the outcomes or products of the process may be lost or not achieved at all. As will be discussed, setting an inappropriate exercise or physical activity programme may precipitate failure, whereas a well-designed programme may lead to a change in lifestyle.

Self-efficacy in exercise programmes

Feelings of confidence in one's own abilities in the exercise setting are thought to arise from several principal sources:

- previous performance attainment in exercise settings,
- copying of others by imitation and modelling,
- verbal and social persuasion,
- judgements of own physiological states in an exercise situation.[20]

Each of these sources has an impact on efficacy expectations and subsequently on the thoughts, emotions and behaviours of the exerciser;[47] therefore, each should be addressed by the exercise professional.

Performance attainment

The self-confidence which is based on successful personal experiences is thought to be an especially powerful source, as success increases confidence and failure reduces confidence.[48] Previous personal attainment and to which factors the individual attributes previous success or failure will be strong influences on efficacy expectation. The situation in which previous experiences occurred may also be a factor.[5]

If the client is currently inactive, they will think about their most recent experience of exercise. This may have been a negative experience and strong unfavourable perceptions about physical activity in general may be apparent. These perceptions may include feelings of boredom, incompetence and embarrassment and may have affected or shaped the person's behaviour since they last participated. A good example of this is the child that is not as gifted in sports as others. They may have been ridiculed at school because of their inability to perform skills well and thus rejected all physical activity in order to avoid the negative experience of feeling incompetent and embarrassed.

Individual experience and perceptions

Exercise can be based on eliciting positive feelings by encouraging success early in the programme. This success may be based on wearing comfortable clothes, making social contacts or by reaching pre-set goals, such as the number of attendances and the ability to achieve the tasks set in the programme. In fact, anything which will fuel the efficacy expectations is essential.

Early success is important, as it will increase confidence and may increase self-esteem, whereas failure may reinforce a lack of self-esteem and confidence.

If a client perceives failure or has not enjoyed a previous attempt at exercising, the adviser can try to establish why and avoid any recurrence of those circumstances.

From the authors' personal experience of delivering cardiac rehabilitation exercise, the client's last experience of formal physical activity/exercise may have been a treadmill exercise stress test which only ends when a person has reached a symptom-limited or volitional maximum. This whole experience can be very frightening and negative, as by definition it ends with some form of failure and/or discomfort.

Some education about how exercise does not have to feel this way, alongside reinforcement of positive elements of activity, a sense of mastery and that exercise can be an enjoyable event in itself, may prove invaluable to developing efficacy expectation and behaviour.

There is support in the research for the view that success on the first attempt leads to an increased likelihood of trying again[47] and that increased self-confidence leads to increased effort and persistence. For this reason, the programme elements of frequency, intensity, mode and duration should be established to ensure a feeling of success.

Modelling

For similar reasons, inviting clients to an exercise session prior to their own attendance, where similar people ('participant' models) are exercising, can provide a view of 'success' with which they can associate. This success can be reinforced for the individual when they begin. The vicarious experience of seeing others exercising without any harmful consequences, but with positive consequences, can develop an expectation for their own improvement and ultimately success. The client may wish to imitate what they have seen if they perceive the model as similar, in age, sex, condition, weight, etc., to themselves. Seeing a young, fit instructor demonstrating the programme may not be as reassuring to the 70-year-old heart bypass patient or overweight 50 year old, as seeing similar others performing the exercise tasks.

The exercise professional should be aware that in a group situation some people may perceive success to be when they have achieved more than another in the group. Matching against other individuals is likely to lead to either boredom or failure, both of which may result in dropout. There is no requirement for this type of competitive comparison in health-related exercise. Regular consultation with an exercise professional could highlight the use of feelings of well-being or self-mastery rather than other reference points such as heart rate at a particular walking speed.[20]

Persuasion

Using verbal or social persuasion is probably going to be fairly weak in effect when compared with the other influencing factors of self-efficacy. The perception of the potential cost and benefits of exercise influence whether a person begins and maintains exercise. This will be discussed later in this chapter. The client may be encouraged, and self-efficacy/confidence increased, by highlighting their achievements. This may be done at each session and reinforced at any follow-up consultation sessions. Talking to oneself positively may also be effective, e.g. 'Yes, I can get to the exercise centre', or 'Yes, I will walk to work, rather than take the car'.

Judgement of physiological states

A person may perceive there to be some form of subjective 'threat' from the exercise situation, such as being watched by others. This may lead to negative emotional arousal. The level of emotional arousal apparent may be measured by heart rate, rating of perceived exertion and other physiological responses. Each individual and group of people is likely to differ in what threat they see from exercise, but if the level of arousal to the threat can be reduced, the perception of self-efficacy will be increased.

The concept of self-efficacy does seem to be an important one for the exercise professional, and self-efficacy theory supports exercise and physical activity being aimed, at least initially, at the promotion of the behaviour, i.e. the participation process rather than the outcome goals and expectations. This suggests a move away from what are still the traditional outcome-based programmes. The process of developing the behaviour must precede, but may lead to, the product or outcome.

This is particularly relevant in England, as the Health Education Authority[49] is promoting physical activity and outcome expectations in terms of health risk reduction and the intrinsic benefits of exercise, as opposed to what might generally be called 'fitness' improvements.

It has been found that self-efficacy correlates strongly with the exercise behaviour of adults and a person's belief that they are able to participate regularly in a structured exercise. As such, self-efficacy seems to be very important.[50] Exercise Professionals should thus incorporate the means for increasing self-efficacy into programmes in order that the chances of exercise behaviour development and adherence will be improved.

The following practical measures are recommended:[51]

1. Set realistic goals.
2. Set a progression of task difficulty (will appeal to person who wants to meet a challenge).
3. Physically aid progressive tasks though 'participant modelling'.
4. Avoid any situations where the person is vulnerable until confidence is built (educational programme may be required to reduce negative stereotyping of certain activities for particular groups).
5. Give feedback. It has been found that women in particular require immediate and objective feedback.
6. Use positive reinforcement, reward mastery attempts, provide positive and appropriate role models. Respected role models who do not communicate disapproval of involvement in physical activity are important for women.
7. Use good communication techniques, e.g. self-talk and praise, anxiety-reducing techniques.

Negative psychological aspects of physical activity and exercise

So far, this chapter has focused on the potential for positive changes in mental well-being as a result of being involved in physical activity and exercise. Exercise has, however, also been associated with some negative problem behaviours, such as exercise dependence and eating disorders.[52] Several terms have been used for those individuals that have become 'exercise dependent',[53] including 'committed' and 'dedicated',[54] 'addicted',[55] 'obligated' and 'fanatical',[56] and 'exercise abusers'.[57]

'Addiction' and 'dependency' may be points on a continuum,[58] but equally they may also represent the same state.[56] There is currently much debate about the use of terminology. Regardless of which label is chosen to describe this *state*, the dependency on exercise could gradually occur with a steady growth in the amount of exercise being performed. The proposed diagnostic criteria for 'exercise dependency' are shown below:[53]

(a) Narrowing of repertoire leading to a stereotyped pattern of exercise with a regular schedule once or more daily.
(b) Giving the individual increasing priority to exercise over other daily activities.
(c) Increased tolerance to the amount of exercise performed over the years.
(d) Withdrawal symptoms related to a disorder of mood following the cessation of the exercise schedule.
(e) Relief or avoidance of withdrawal symptoms by further exercise.
(f) Subjective awareness of a compulsion to exercise.
(g) Rapid reinstatement of the previous pattern of exercise and withdrawal symptoms after a period of abstinence.

Associated features
(h) Either the individual continues to exercise despite a serious physical disorder known to be caused, aggravated or prolonged by exercise and is advised as such by a health professional, or the individual has arguments or difficulties with his/her partner, family, friends or occupation.
(i) Self-inflicted loss of weight by dieting as a means towards improving performance.

Eventually the dependent individual will put exercise before all other aspects of their life, including family, work and social life. Assuming that they will not stop or reduce the level of exercise, regardless of advice given by doctors, exercise professionals, family, friends and colleagues, the individual may find that work, family and social problems arise, as well as physical injuries.

When the individual is incapable of making choices, an addiction exists and awareness may have been lost, involvement in other activities hindered, self-esteem lowered, and the predictable activity may no longer give pleasure.[58] When these individuals are unable to participate in their chosen activity because of illness or holidays, etc., they may develop withdrawal symptoms, including increased levels of depression.[55]

Exercise dependency may be categorized as being primary or secondary. If the exercise is an end in itself and weight loss or dietary changes are to help performance, this is known as primary exercise dependence. Exercise dependence may be secondary if it is due to an eating disorder such as bulimia nervosa or anorexia nervosa, where the aim is to use the exercise to help maintain weight loss.

Individuals dependent on exercise share many of the characteristics of those that are eating disordered:[59]

- dietary faddism,
- controlled calorie consumption,
- low body weight,
- high physical activity,
- high levels of body awareness.

These negative consequences of exercise and physical activity would normally only occur in response to a training stimulus that is more frequent, longer in duration and more intense than is required to promote health or fitness.[60]

Staleness and overtraining in athletes is another possible negative consequence of exercise and has been found to lead to behavioural and psychological problems such as sleep disturbances, emotional distress and depression.[61]

Exercise programming and monitoring should be tailored to maximize the psychological benefits while being aware of the possible negative outcomes.

Stress

Stress is probably the most commonly used term to describe a variety of psychological and physiological conditions. It is fair to say that stress is a major health concern for this and the next century, as it has been associated with a number of illnesses, such as coronary heart disease and suppression of the immune system. Stressors, the reasons for the stress response, are varied and depend on the individual's perception and circumstances. For instance, a client may feel that attending an exercise centre is a situation which is stressful to them. The response to the stressor will be based on a release of various hormones, which lead the client to experience physiological responses such as increased heart rate and blood pressure.

Commonly known as the 'fight or flight' response, this may be a very useful response for a caveman escaping from a sabre-toothed tiger, when all of his body systems have to be switched on immediately to save his life! But if there is no physical situation in which to vent this response, it can be very unhealthy, particularly if the stress is experienced over a long period of time.

Activity and exercise may provide the opportunity to 'release' stress psychologically and physiologically, whether the stressor is from work, driving, personal problems, etc., therefore aiding health.

It is beyond the scope of this chapter to discuss all aspects of stress in full, but there are several informative and entertaining texts which examine this subject and give it the coverage it so apparently deserves. One such, is Robert Sapolsky's *Why Zebras Don't Get Ulcers*.[62]

In general, when promoting long-term health-related exercise, unnecessary stressors should be avoided, to make exercise a relatively stress-free and enjoyable experience. In this way the stress-minimizing effects of exercise may be maintained.

A summary of the some of the main effects of exercise and physical activity on mental well-being are shown below:

- exercise has a small beneficial effect on anxiety and reactivity to stress,
- exercise has a moderate to large beneficial effect on mild to moderate depression,
- exercise has a moderately favourable effect on psychological well-being,

- exercise may be associated with positive changes in selected aspects of personality – psychological adjustment and cognitive functioning,
- a few individuals are compulsive about exercise; such compulsive behaviour may be unhealthy,
- the environment of sport and exercise has the potential for making a significant positive impact on participants' prosocial behaviours, although the current programmes have both positive and negative effects.

How physical activity may improve mental health – the mechanisms

Having made a link between exercise and mental well-being, researchers have investigated the mechanisms responsible for any psychological changes. The mechanisms described below can be categorized as being of a physiological or a psychosocial nature and they may work alone or together to produce effects such as reduced levels of depression and anxiety and improved mood (Figure 3.3).

Endorphin hypothesis

The release of naturally occurring opiate-like substances known as endorphins is an example of a possible physiological response. Perhaps the most commonly known of the mechanisms involves the chemical release of the brain's endorphin, leading to a feeling of improved well-being following a bout of exercise. This is sometimes referred to as a 'fix' of endorphins which leads to a 'runner's high'. Another common, unproven, belief is that it the need for this fix which leads to an 'exercise addiction'.

The endorphin hypothesis is, however, only one of several possible mechanisms which are thought may be the link between exercise and

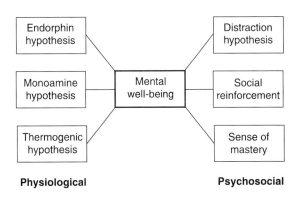

Figure 3.3 Mechanisms of improved mental well-being from physical activity and exercise.

improvement in mental health and although probably the least well supported, there is some evidence for this mechanism.[63, 64]

The monoamine hypothesis

Monoamines are chemicals such as norepinephrine, serotonin and dopamine, which act to transport nerve impulses. The monoamine hypothesis is based on the the assumption that the neurobiological actions of exercise could be similar to those of drug treatments. Therefore, that the improved effect which is associated with exercise is explained by changes in one or all of the circulating monoamines.[65,66]

The thermogenic hypothesis

The thermogenic hypothesis is simply based on the effect of warmth or heat and is reasonably supported by research evidence showing that anxiety in the form of muscle tension may be reduced following a sauna or a hot shower.[28] During exercise we experience an increase in core body temperature and it is possible that it is this which produces the therapeutic effect, which may last for several hours after the session. The intensity of the exercise may mediate or determine the effect.

The effect may be due to the reduced muscle tension, the release of chemical substances which produce fever (pyrogens), or because the increased temperature influences the release, synthesis or uptake of the monoamines.

Distraction theory

The time required to take part in exercise may allow for a 'time out' effect or a distraction from anxiety and everyday stresses, much as relaxation might.[29] It has been found that although the mental health benefits of exercise and relaxation are quantitatively similar, the effect from exercise lasts somewhat longer and is therefore qualitatively different.

The 'distraction'[29] effect is encouraging for the promotion of exercise adherence, as it allows the suggestion that the process of being involved in physical activity is at least as important as the product.

Distraction or 'diversion' is an example of a possible psychosocial mechanism for the improvement of mental health.[67]

Social reinforcement

The exercise adviser and other clients are able to provide social reinforcement[68] in the form of attention, praise and encouragement. A client receiving what they perceive to be positive verbal feedback and social interaction may have their exercise behaviour strengthened. The concept of reinforcement of behaviour will be discussed further later in the chapter. As positive reinforcement leads to a strengthening of the behaviour, comments and terminology which could be interpreted as negative or patronizing should be avoided. Tone of voice and physical gestures/body signals are also important to consider.

An example of positive reinforcement for the client involved in the exercise 'process' is 'Well done, you have attended despite not having the car today' or, on the basis of improved function (product), 'Well done, you are now walking 1 kph faster and for 3 minutes longer than 3 weeks ago'.

It is often useful for partnerships or groups of clients to encourage each other through the early stages of the programme in particular. The 'buddy' system is a very useful tool for the exercise professional, who can also stimulate informal 'buddying' between exercisers by creating an atmosphere and situation in which social interaction is possible. The exercise professional in this instance could be considered to act as a catalyst for social reinforcement. Individual differences must be considered by the exercise professional, as each client is likely to respond more positively to various means of reinforcement.

Sense of mastery

Setting the elements of exercise programmes to allow the client some perception of success and achievement may promote a feeling that they are able to perform the required tasks. This may be the tasks established while actually exercising, or the task of exhibiting the behaviour, such as attending twice per week, etc. They can then experience the sense that they have 'mastered' the required activity.[27,68] To enable this, the exercise professional may have to consider a trade-off between physiological and psychological improvements. The initial programme may not be of sufficient intensity to have a large effect on factors of fitness (see Chapters 1, 2 and 7), but if the client participates regularly, partly due to 'mastery', the process of fitness is being established. In time, the client and the exercise professional may decide to progress the programme to a higher intensity. It should be noted that health benefits may be derived from low levels of exercise intensity, if the activity takes place regularly.[69]

A sense of mastery is one of several feelings which are anticipated as outcomes of exercise participation, which can also provide some motivation for continuing the activity.[44] In order to incorporate the important element of mastery into exercise programmes, it should be ensured that the patient is well instructed in techniques and that no element of the programme will be beyond their capabilities.

An example would be that balance is often difficult on a treadmill; therefore, handrails could be used initially. When the handrails are no longer required by the client, this may present them with a 'sense of mastery'.

Summary of mechanisms

Any one or all of the mechanisms discussed may be responsible for the improvements in mental health and well-being which are associated with exercise and physical activity. So far there is no consensus as to the relative importance of each of the proposed mechanisms. It remains to be established whether psychological changes occur as a result of non-specific effects such as 'diversion', 'social reinforcement' or 'experience of mastery', or to specific physiological responses to exercise stress, such as the effects of substances like endorphins on the central nervous system.[70]

From a practical viewpoint it is emphasized that the question is whether or not exercise serves as an effective form of treatment irrespective of its *modus operandi* (method).[71] From the epidemiological, physiological and psychological evidence presented in this book, there is one point which is abundantly clear and should be the guiding light for all exercise and activity programming ... however well-constructed a programme may be, whether it is designed for an elite athlete or the most sedentary members of our population, there can be no beneficial consequences without taking part in physical activity – *participation is the key*!

Part III   Developing the 'exercise habit'

It is apparent that a client can experience a great many positive benefits from merely participating in regular exercise, particularly that which is aerobic in nature. Regardless of this, many clients will not complete a programme of exercise and will not incorporate physical activity into their lifestyle. As has just been emphasized, if the client does not take part in the 'process', there will be no 'product'.

A most challenging aspect for the exercise professional is the development of the clients' long-term adherence to exercise and physical activity behaviour or, in other words, the positive exercise habit.

In order that a client can move towards an active lifestyle and begin or maintain a programme of exercise, the exercise professional should be aware of the factors that may precede and/or support the behaviour and how these factors are thought to fit into the general scheme of exercise behaviour. Programmes can then be tailored to fit each individual client, depending on their particular circumstances, and the likelihood of adherence increased.

Adherence to exercise

Several terms related to exercise adherence are used in this text. Definitions are as follows:[72]

- *Adherence*. Fulfilment of predetermined goals, i.e. if the goal of an exercise programme is 5 times per week for 30 minutes and this goal is met on 20 out of 25 weeks, adherence is 80%.
- *Compliance*. Adherence and compliance are often used interchangeably, although sometimes compliance is used in medical circumstances, such as compliance to a course of drugs.
- *Short-term adherence*. This indicates adherence during a programme which lasts for a specific time period in weeks/months, etc.

● *Dropouts.* Those who discontinue participation in an exercise programme. Some will, however, continue to exercise (or take part in physical activity) on their own; therefore, the term must be distinguished from adherence. As already mentioned, it is possible for a person to 'drop out' of an exercise programme but continue to adhere to a physicaly active lifestyle.

Despite the great many positive reasons for being physically active, up to 50% of individuals who start an aerobic exercise programme will drop out within the first 6 months.[3,72] Although this figure is very high, dropouts from exercise are probably no more frequent than for drug or psychotherapies.[11]

It has been noted that dropout rates from exercise programmes are higher in aerobic activities than those which are less aerobic, and that adherence in clinical populations does not differ much from other populations.[15]

Despite the previously stated dropout rate of 50%, research has shown that adherence rates of 85–95% are attainable for properly supervised exercise programmes.[72,73] As rates as high as this are possible and it is known that to maintain the benefits of physical activity the exercise must be continued, then effective approaches to encouraging the maintenance of exercise programmes are needed.

For example, a client with an anxiety disorder may associate increased exercise and 'normal' symptoms of exercise stress, such as sweating, with increased anxiety. To prevent the patient dropping out of the programme to avoid this unpleasant experience, the programme could be adapted to be of lower intensity so that the client feels that the exercise is comfortable to them. The ratings of perceived exertion (RPE) scales are a useful tool for this. The client may then feel capable of achieving the programme and a 'sense of mastery' may evolve, leading to longer term adherence.

It is clear that an overall explanation of exercise adherence is complex and those who may be able to derive the greatest benefit from adhering to exercise may be the least willing to adhere due to the 'weight' of all the other factors.[73] Adherence should not be viewed as an all-or-none phenomenon, but a process that may change throughout the cycle.[69]

There may be many factors which cause changes in adherence. Those which reduce or prevent the initiation or adherence to exercise can be considered to be barriers, and may be categorized as real or perceived. The key challenge to the exercise professional is to examine all of the known barriers and aid the client in deciding a course of action to break them down. This concept is discussed later in the chapter and illustrated in Table 3.1.

Behaviour – cues and consequences

Behaviour may be affected by the signals, cues and circumstances which precede it (antecedents) as well as the positive or negative outcomes (consequences) which follow it. A red light is the antecedent to stopping the car, hopefully avoiding an accident which is a positive consequence. There are various theories which address these areas and they are concerned with how and why a person might 'learn' to behave in a particular way, for instance learning to be physically active.

Learning can be thought of as using past experiences to form a permanent or relatively permanent change in a behaviour. Structured exercise programmes may provide a platform to begin the activity process which can then be carried through into a 'normal' lifestyle. As a client gains more positive 'past experiences' to reward their activity efforts, the more likely it becomes that a relatively permanent change in exercise behaviour will occur.

Cues for exercise

The time, the place and the other people involved could all be considered to be cues that may increase the stimulus for the exercise behaviour. In other words a cue is a 'spark' that may lead to doing or not doing some exercise. From the authors' observation, experiencing a heart attack often becomes a very strong cue to becoming more physically active. Patients often become fitter, happier and even healthier after a course of rehabilitation than they were prior to the heart attack.

Another example, for instance, is by arranging to meet a partner or friend at the same place and time prior to each exercise session, the chances of successfully attending the session are increased. Eventually, the client may learn to associate a particular place or time of the week or day with exercise. Obvious examples of behavioural antecedents are being in pub as the cue for having a drink or a cigarette, or the smell of the fish and chip shop providing enough of stimulus for you to buy fish and chips. Although over-simplistic, it perhaps seems obvious to suggest that if you did not want to drink, smoke or eat fish and chips, then you should avoid going to the pub and walking past the fish and chip shop.

In the context of exercise, we want to encourage cues that may stimulate the exhibition of the exercise behaviour while dealing with cues that discourage the desired behaviour. What may at first appear to be an excuse for not doing exercise may in fact be due to other, strong cues to exhibit another 'competing' behaviour'. This can arise in a formal exercise centre setting itself, by the lure of a sauna or a conversation with a friend in the coffee bar. Competing cues may also, and often do, arise in other situations.

Getting into the car after work may be a cue for going home to dinner rather than driving to an exercise centre. Eating dinner and exercise are, in this case, competing behaviours. Identifying these cues will aid the development of interventions to modify or avoid the stimulus so that it does not lead to an inability to exercise or the breakdown of an established pattern of behaviour. For example, getting a lift to work so that the only way home is to walk, or taking exercise clothing to work, may provide a stronger cue to do some exercise than other cues provide to go home for tea.

Competing cues can be manipulated or even eliminated by preplanning likely situations and providing the client with an alternative response or a substitute to a particular cue that would lead to non-performance of the desired exercise behaviour.

Consistently taking regular exercise following a particular 'cue situation' will increase the power of that cue to elicit the response of exercise. In contrast to this, the removal of the cues for exercise, such as at the end of the programme period, will reduce the chances of the exercise response. Careful planning to encourage cues outside the normal exercise programme cues can help to overcome this problem and lead to increased adherence.

Consequences and rewards of exercise

When a session of exercise is followed by a positive outcome or reward, the likelihood of the behaviour being repeated in future or increased. Positive outcomes may be in many forms, such as how enjoyable the session was, how someone feels better for having done some exercise, or the perception that they are improving an aspect of their fitness.

Conversely, a negative outcome may act to decrease future occurrence of the behaviour. The importance of enjoyment to exercise behaviour should not be underestimated.[39] If the session is not enjoyable, or perceived as being too hard or too easy, the exerciser may feel that they would rather have spent the time doing something else. The lack of enjoyment may also be due to a secondary situation, e.g. finding a space to park the car. Especially so when it is left completely to their own volition, such as following the conclusion of their programme.

An exerciser can be encouraged to develop physically active behaviours if they feel that there is some reward for their efforts. Often this may be derived from attaining a pre-set goal.

Rewards

'Extrinsic' rewards are usually considered to be tangible and may be in many forms: a tick on an attendance card; a tee-shirt for having completed the course; praise from the instructor. Other forms of reward are 'intrinsic' or personal to each individual and may include such things as feeling good for having attended or the joy of being active for its own sake. Extrinsic rewards are a good way of encouraging a behaviour when a client begins a programme as long as they perceive the reward positively. If they feel that the reward is not worth the effort or time spent gaining it, then the effect is likely to lead to a decrease in exercise behaviour.

Over time, as the client begins to appreciate and emphasize the pleasurable consequences of exercising, reliance on external rewards can and should be gradually removed. Exercise may then become a 'self-reinforcing' behaviour and it is likely that the behaviour will persist.[75] To this end, the variety of activities offered within the exercise prescription should provide for a choice of exercise which has interest and appeal to the individual. The consequences of exercise will have a powerful effect on manipulating the behaviour positively or negatively and each individual must be considered separately.

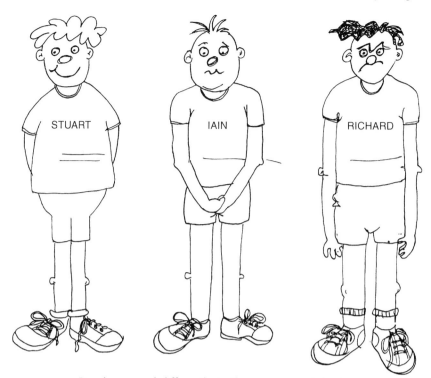

People respond differently to the same rewards/praise

The following example (and accompanying sketch) illustrate how the instructor can influence future behaviour:

- Stuart may perceive praise from the instructor to be a very positive external reward for his efforts and the chances of him repeating the exercise behaviour are strengthened.
- Iain is less outgoing than Stuart and may be embarrassed at being singled out from the group for praise and considers this to be a very negative consequence and is less likely to repeat the exercise behaviour.
- Richard does not really like the instructor and considers the praise to be patronising and also considers this to be negative. He too is less likely to repeat the behaviour, and therefore praise needs to be altered to suit the client's personality.

There are other, very powerful social reinforcers such as family and friends who may all influence the behaviour positively or negatively. Engaging the support of such people to provide positive comments and responses to the client's efforts to exercise would also greatly enhance the chances for longer term adherence. Most cardiac rehabilitation programmes engage family education and awareness sessions and provide leaflets and posters to aid the families in understanding the condition and their part in long-term recovery.

Similar strategies can successfully be employed for non-clinical groups by providing social events, information leaflets and posters. If the information presented is selected based on each client's individual needs, then this process can be effective.

The local press can have a very big impact on the community and shaping its knowledge and understanding of exercise. For example, the exercise professional can provide information to the press in the form of articles or radio interviews. By incorporating projects or people that the community are likely to be aware of, or will affect them, the information is likely to be more readily accepted.

Barriers to exercise and physical activity participation

However much a client may wish to become physically active, there may be factors that stand between them and the development of a new behaviour. Barriers which prevent a person from taking exercise may be real or there may be a subjective perception that a barrier exists.

A 'real' barrier may be a lack of money, a lack of facilities, or even a cultural barrier. 'Perceived' barriers are felt by the client whether or not they are viewed by others as posing a problem. If the client feels that there is a barrier, then this must be dealt with. Perceived barriers are believed to have a stronger influence than real barriers, because most exercise behaviour is under a person's own control.

Barriers to exercise may relate to past experiences or preconceptions, which can sometimes be overcome with some educational input from the exercise professional.

The Allied Dunbar National Fitness Survey[74] examined such barriers in the UK and categorized them as shown in Table 3.1 (see also accompanying sketch). Also shown are the most popular reasons for not being physically active within each category. The table provides examples of both real and perceived barriers which will face the exercise

Table 3.1 Barriers to physical activity. (Adapted from Health Education Authority[74])

Physical barriers	Emotional barriers	Motivational barriers	Time barriers	Availability barriers
I have an injury or disability that stops me	I'm not the sporty type	I need to rest and relax in my spare time	I haven't got the time	There is no one to do it with
I'm too fat	I'm too shy or embarrassed	I haven't got the energy	I don't have time because of my work	I can't afford it
My health is not good enough	I might get injured or damage my health	I'd never keep it up	I've got very young children to look after	There are no suitable facilities nearby
I'm too old		I don't enjoy physical activity		I haven't got the right clothes or equipment

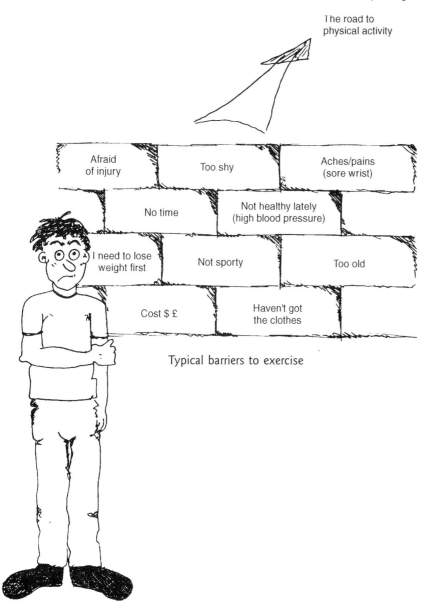

Typical barriers to exercise

professional. Dealing with these barriers is very much a matter for the individuals concerned, but some common situations can be examined.

Lack of time

Lack of time is an often quoted reason for not being physically active and if a client suggests that they have no time at all for any exercise, then it would at first seem that the door has been slammed firmly shut. The exercise professional must establish whether this is a real or perceived barrier and whether or not it is a true barrier or merely some form of defence mechanism to prevent the client having to tell you that they really do not want to be physically active. In the latter case, the interventions aimed at clients in a pre-contemplation stage of behaviour change could be employed. See stages of behaviour change near the end of this chapter for further discussion.

If there is real lack of time, there are several options. Education about the importance and the benefits of being physically active may encourage the client to look at their timetable with a view to identifying any slots where the important activity can occur. This may be done by keeping a diary of all daily activities as well as through discussion. It may well be that the lack of time is a time management or perceived problem.

If no time slots can be found to set aside for physical activity or exercise, there may be means to incorporate activity into the current lifestyle. For instance, more walking in the office, perhaps by walking to see someone rather than telephoning them, delivering memos in person rather than by internal post, or taking short breaks to have a walk around the building, may be perceived as being of benefit. This may then lead to further development of the exercise behaviour.

Emotional barriers

The comment that a person is not physically active because they are 'not the sporty type' demonstrates a basic lack of understanding of physical activity and possibly reflects that a person has had some previous negative experiences which they now associate with any exercise and physical activity. As it is a person's perception and knowledge which drive this type of comment, identifying activities in which the client already engages can be of use. If they see that they are already physically active in some way, because they garden regularly or enjoy walking, their perception may change. Use of the terminology which best fits the client may encourage participation, e.g. the term 'exercise' may be perceived as being all sport-type activities, but encouraging an increase in 'physical activity' may not carry any negative preconception – after all, we are all physically active to some degree. Awareness of the differences in definitions may also help.

Motivational barriers

Educating the client that physical activity and exercise can be relaxing and can increase energy levels may help in the process of breaking down motivational barriers. If the client has positive experiences when they begin to be more physically active, then future motivation to participate is likely to be enhanced.

Most people enjoy some form of physical activity. The exercise professional has to identify this. Emphasizing another aspect of the benefit of being more active may provide more motivation. For instance, a grandparent may feel that they enjoy playing with their grandchildren, but soon get worn out. Emphasizing that they would be more able to enjoy this activity if they were generally more active may motivate them. Simply pointing out that some types of play with grandchildren is physically active may remove the barrier of all activity being seen as unenjoyable.

Availability barriers

There may genuinely be little in the way of accessible facilities for the client. The exercise professional can design exercise that can be performed without formal facilities and that will be of minimum financial cost. For example, walking is an activity that does not require any specialist facility or clothing, other than an appropriate pair of shoes, in most cases.

The idea of advice about physical activity for health is addressed further in Chapter 7. The exercise professional can help the client to realize the social opportunities of exercise and physical activity. It is possible that one of these is insurmountable; for example, due to cultural differences an Asian woman may not be able to attend a formal programme run by a male instructor, but would be able to pursue a programme of physical activity on her own.

Beliefs and attitudes about physical activity and exercise

Although the mechanisms for exercise participation are by no means fully understood, the beliefs and attitudes of the client may be important to the exercise behaviour. The health belief model (HBM)[76] proposes that it is the individual's perception of the threat to their health and the perception that a recommended preventative action will reduce the threat.

If a common GP referral scenario is assumed: a person reads a health promotion leaflet informing them of the health risks of their being physically inactive, and they also feel that their age, sex and race are complementary factors of risk. There may now be a perception of the threat of disease, which may motivate the person to consult their GP who may present the benefits of physical activity as well as helping to remove any initial real or perceived barriers to the first contact with an exercise professional, perhaps by booking the first appointment for them.

Following the HBM, if the person now holds the belief that exercise removes a perceived threat from disease, and the barriers have been addressed, it is likely that they will become physically active.

Further research is required to show whether the HBM is appropriate for the study of exercise behaviour. The intrinsic motivation derived from the pleasure of exercising, rather than the extrinsic health rewards, may be the force that motivates people, rather than the fear of disease.

An accepted definition of attitude is that it is 'a latent or nonobservable, complex, but relatively stable behavioural disposition reflecting both direction and intensity of feeling toward a particular object'.[77] As illustrated by the definition itself, attitude is an apparently very complex area of understanding. In simple terms, attitude to exercise can be considered to be constructed from a person's beliefs about the likely outcomes of being physically active, and whether the outcomes will be of value to the individual (socially, physically, psychologically).

The theory of reasoned action[78] and the theory of planned behaviour[79] were developed to predict and understand behaviour. Both models suggest that a person's intention to be physically active will partly depend upon their attitude towards exercise and physical activity, and that a person's intention to exercise will mediate the actual behaviour.

The beliefs of 'significant others', such as a partner, other family, peers, etc., may affect the intention to exercise. This depends on the degree to which the client wishes to comply with these beliefs. The client may or may not be easily influenced by others.

The relative importance that the client applies to the attitudes and beliefs of others is also considered in these theories. A person's own attitude is likely to be more important than the beliefs of others, as most people believe that it is their own responsibility whether to exercise or not.

The theory of planned behaviour was developed in response to criticism of the theory of reasoned action. It includes an element of 'perceived behavioural control' as well as attitude, and the beliefs of others as a mediator of the intention to exercise and ultimately to actually take part in activity.

The perceived behavioural control reflects a person's perception of how difficult or easy it will be to perform the behaviour. This will, in turn, reflect on barriers to exercise such as existing obstacles and negative past experiences.

The process of changing exercise behaviour

Much of the research into behaviours such as smoking and drug taking suggests that successful behaviour change involves a process of steps or stages before lifetime change can occur.

The stages of change model (transtheoretical model)[80–82] is promoted in England by the Health Education Authority in the provision of behaviour change training for health professionals (Figure 3.4). This model provides the exercise professional with a tool for helping people overcome the 'barriers' to a physically active lifestyle.

In practical terms, there is a key difference between using the model for promoting physical activity, as opposed to other 'healthy behaviours', such as smoking cessation. The focus is on enabling a person to add positive exercise behaviour to their lives, rather than take away a negative health behaviour like smoking.

In essence, the model promotes the modification of behaviour by examining biological, psychological and environmental factors and developing interventions matched to the specific stage of change the client is currently at. The exercise professional can then enable and support the client in making the changes necessary to maintain the process of exercise and physical activity.

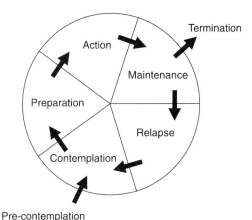

Pre-contemplation

Figure 3.4 The Basic Stages of Change model (transtheoretical model) promoted by the Health Education Authority in England.[80 – 82]

It is probably too simplistic to discuss the exercise process as being a single behaviour, as there may be several behaviours to be modified and developed before the desired behaviour is achieved. For example, if the client wishes to exercise on two evenings per week when they would otherwise be at the pub, their social behaviour has to be modified to allow the exercise behaviour to develop. If they prefer to take some exercise at lunchtime, their eating behaviours may have to be modified. It seems that the process of exercise is likely to be a chain of behaviours.[3]

The diagram in Figure 3.4 is a representation of how the client may move from one stage to another.

The exercise professional must determine which stage their client is at and apply the interventions relevant to that particular stage. In this way the client can gradually move towards a change in exercise behaviour which will last a lifetime. Although the diagram shows only arrows moving in one direction, it is possible for the client to move forwards and backwards through the stages.

As is shown in the illustration, there are generally considered to be seven stages:

1. Pre-contemplation.
2. Contemplation.
3. Preparation.
4. Action.
5. Maintenance.
6. Relapse.
7. Termination.

Pre-contemplators – not interested in changing 'risky' lifestyle

People in the pre-contemplation stage are not currently exercising and have no intention to do so in the near future. They are not even contemplating any change. This is a stable stage and individuals may remain in it anything from 6 months to 2 years if interventions are employed, possibly for life if not.

As the client has no intention of changing, using 'pushy' techniques in an attempt to force them to change is unlikely to be effective. If the exercise professional sees a client in this stage, they may not have rejected the idea of exercise outright; after all, they are at least talking or have attended an appointment.

It may be difficult at the first meeting for the exercise professional to gain the information they require. The client will not have had the opportunity to develop a personal relationship with the professional and may not feel that they can place their trust in a relative stranger. They may have adopted the attitude that what they do is their own business and that if they did discuss exercise, they may be judged or criticized. Any such comments should be avoided by the exercise professional.

Interventions

At this stage the current health status of the client should be established. The exercise professional can then raise the issue of physical activity and provide awareness and educational information.

Asking the client about their current exercise knowledge can aid discussion and illuminate any fallacies or gaps there may be and provide information about past experiences of exercise, which may well have been negative.

A physically inactive person may believe that only fit people can exercise or that you have to get hot, sweaty and out of breath to gain any benefit. Awareness and education about the true facts and how activity can be very enjoyable if the right form is selected, alongside basic advice about how the first step can be taken, is very important.

It should be remembered that although information about risk prevention may be given, promoting exercise via the fear of risks to health may not be as useful as presenting the more obviously positive factors such as enjoyment, rewards and social interaction.

Contemplators – thinking about change

These are clients that have an intention to become more physically active in the near future, but are currently putting off the change. They may already have reasons for considering exercise and physical activity, perhaps because they have become aware of how beneficial it may be for their health or because they think they may enjoy it. It is likely that the identification of 'significant life events' such as myocardial infarction (heart attack) or the presence of high blood pressure being recognized, may precipitate contemplation of healthy behaviours such as physical activity.

This is a relatively stable stage and the client may stay in it for up to 2 years before starting to change exercise behaviour.

Interventions

Clients in this stage should be encouraged to weigh up the pros and cons of physical activity, while considering the health risks if they are not active. These risks are outlined in Chapter 2.

Any harm that already exists to their health, such as high blood pressure, excessive fat or anxiety, can be recorded, without being judgemental. This provides baseline information against which a client can be measured in future.

All of the concerns a client may have about making changes should be discussed sympathetically, regardless of how trivial or illogical they may at first seem. It is the client's perception which is important, and what may seem a relatively minor concern to the exercise professional may be the single biggest barrier to the client starting exercise.

A clinical example is that of a patient following a heart attack (myocardial infarction). They may have a perception that they should not be physically active, when in fact such patients are able to exercise within the first 10 days of the event. The contemplation stage in these cases may be very short, but the necessary interventions should still occur. Solutions and information may then be offered to help reduce any existing fears.

This is a time when some of the barriers preventing exercise and physical activity can be broached. It should be remembered, however, that other factors of life may be beyond the exercise professional's role. There may be aspects of home and work life that will prevent the move to the next stage until they are seen as less of a priority. The exercise professional may be able to discuss these issues and suggest that other practical assistance is sought. When these issues are less of a priority, the client may be ready to take the next step.

From earlier discussion it has been noted that lack of time is a key reason offered for not being physically active. Asking a client to keep a diary allows the identification of time slots that may be utilized for exercise. It is possible that the 'lack of time' for exercise is not real, but perceived. A diary helps establish the reality, which is often recognized without any prompting from the exercise professional.

Preparation – preparing to change

Clients at this stage are intending to start becoming more physically active in the next month. They may already have started to increase their levels of activity in general.

Preparation is considered an unstable stage, as it may not last very long. Clients are more likely to move on a stage in the near future, than those in the more stable stages such as pre-contemplation and contemplation.

Interventions

The client should receive encouragement and, where possible, barriers to taking the next step should be addressed.

Foreseeable 'traps' or temptations away from the exercise behaviour can be discussed and alternatives suggested. An example would be that in order to go to an exercise centre after work, the client will have to pass his home. After a hard day, when he is feeling hungry and tired, he may be tempted to miss out the exercise and just go home. The exercise professional may suggest driving an alternative route to avoid the risk of temptation or suggest using the distraction of thinking about how good he would feel if he exercised before going home.

The client should also be aware of a choice of alternative activities that suit their particular circumstances and preferences. Some clients will prefer activities that they can do alone, such as cycling, rather than those which require social interaction, such as line dancing. Usually the client has developed a plan to follow when they do make the change.

For long-term behaviour change to occur, clients should have easy alternative ways to meet their needs. If the client lacks social support for the exercise behaviour from friends that she usually meets at the bingo hall, then provision of a friendly exercise group may give the client an easy alternative to meeting her social needs. She will then be less likely to perceive there to be a social cost to being active.

There may still be unresolved barriers of a higher priority to the client than the exercise, and the exercise professional must know when to advise alternative practical help to ease the problem and possibly where this help can be reached. Examples of this kind of problem could be marital difficulties or family illness.

Action – making changes

The client has changed their behaviour within the last 6 months. This is the least stable of all the stages and there is a high risk of relapse.

Good planning in the stages prior to making the change may prevent dropout and or relapse, by planning the activity on the basis of the following 'SMART' mnemonic.[49]

Interventions

Specific objectives – e.g. attend the exercise centre three times per week.
Measurable results – to provide feedback and progression.
Agreement – to ensure that the plan is what suits the client.
Realism – small steps to ensure the client believes the change is possible.
Time scale – when to start and when to review progress.

The exercise professional must provide flexibility in the approach at this stage. If the client finds that attending three times per week is too demanding despite all of the planning, then attendance of twice per week may become the realistic and agreed goal.

This type of change must be handled carefully if it is not to be perceived as a 'failure' on the part of the client, e.g. 'Well done, you were doing no exercise at all and now you are doing two sessions per week'.

Positive reinforcement is essential at all times and may initially be given as an extrinsic reward. Examples of this are earning a free session or an exercise clothing discount after a certain number of sessions. Although almost traditional now, the award of a tee-shirt is generally accepted as a symbol of achievement and acceptance.

Positive support should continue and the intrinsic reward of exercising for its own sake, such as 'feeling better', must be promoted if longer term maintenance is to be achieved.

Maintenance – maintaining changes

Once the client has maintained the physically active behaviour for 6 months they are deemed to be in the maintenance stage. The changes are still taking place and barriers need to be continually addressed. The exercise professional may need to anticipate future barriers, such as sickness, having children, changing work shifts, etc., and provide interventions for such eventualities.

Interventions

Support from the family and the environment is required. Positive changes for the client may be perceived negatively by a member of the family or a friend. Their support would then be withdrawn and may even become a form of sabotage to make exercising difficult. A spouse may feel deprived of the time that exercise is taking away from them. They may also feel that because their partner is becoming more confident, attractive and 'fitter', that the new differences between them are a threat and they will then discourage, sometimes unconsciously, exercise behaviour. Enlisting firm support from the spouse or partner in the earlier stages may reduce the threat from support sabotage.

Further support for the client may be gained from the exercise group or from being paired with a 'buddy' for exercise sessions.

Methods for the avoidance of 'risk' situations which may lead to a decrease in the exercise behaviour can also be readdressed.

Periodical reviews of a client's exercise programme and their response to their 'activity environment' can help to maintain the enjoyment and achievement experiences. By this stage the rewards are likely to be intrinsic and felt to be worth doing for their own sake. Feedback based on the original assessment may be useful for further motivation.

As the client becomes more involved with exercise there may be a tendency to develop a 'more is better' philosophy. This can be discussed and the awareness of injury risk and other negative elements, such as the possibility of family disruption, is highlighted.

Relapse

Relapsing to a non-active state is a normal and expected part of the behaviour change process and some clients may experience several loops around the stages before reaching the goal of the maintenance and termination stages.[4] The mistakes and choices made which led to a relapse can be learned from and planned against to prevent similar relapse at a later date. Planning for return to activity following a 'forced relapse' because of illness or holidays can help prevent a 'full-blown' relapse.

Interventions

The client and the exercise professional can plan and discuss the likelihood of relapse and any high-risk situations where it is foreseen as being a likely outcome. Discussing the possibility of relapse with the client at the outset will lessen any shock and perception of failure, which it is hoped will lessen the negative impact there may be on self-confidence. In fact, the skilful exercise professional can change the perception of relapse to a positive one by reminding the client that having relapsed they are now that much nearer to achieving the physically active behaviour they desire. The client will realise that there is a way back and that they have already achieved a degree of the behaviour.

If the lapse is relatively temporary, it can be prevented from becoming a more complete relapse by concentrating on the next episode of 'good' behaviour rather than by dwelling on the episode of relapse. Dealing with a temporary lapse also begins in earlier planning stages by discussing how to deal with it. For instance, the busy executive may be expected occasionally to miss a planned session because of unexpected work pressure. Rather than thinking about the one session missed in the week, the client can be encouraged to concentrate on the other sessions that are part of the programme. The one missed session should not then become the reason for missing a whole week of the programme.

If the client is in a formal exercise programme, with continual contact with an exercise professional, boredom and social or emotional pressures may be detected and discussed. This is not as simple for independent physical activity programmes, where the client himself would have to recognize situations where there is high risk of relapse and take appropriate action, perhaps by avoiding the situation in the first place.

Alternatives should always be available to allow the client to meet other needs without relapsing. When there is a need for a stressed client to let off a little steam, a good bike ride may perform the same function as sitting alone in the pub may have done in the past.

The cause of any problems always needs to be carefully examined rather just recognizing the symptoms. The symptom may be that exercise is erratic because of personal problems at home. Dealing with the cause may not be within the scope of the exercise professional, but understanding this may allow a re-setting of the exercise goals and a change in the programme direction to prevent complete relapse.

Relapse is not necessarily all or nothing; just because a client has not exercised for a month does not mean that the behaviour has ceased. It does seem that no matter what strategy is applied, the majority of people will relapse at some point. The experiences gained from this should

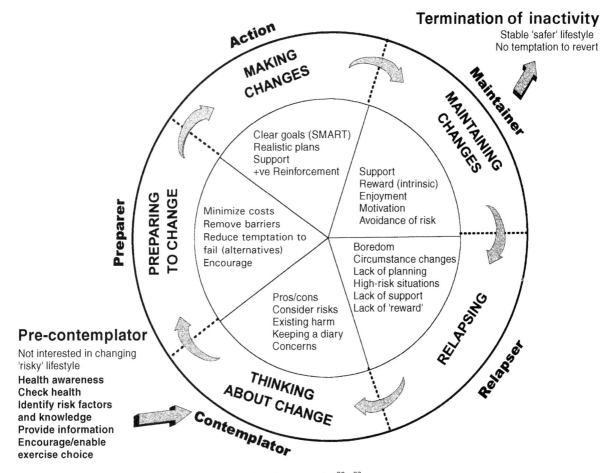

Termination of inactivity
Stable 'safer' lifestyle
No temptation to revert

Maintainer

MAINTAINING CHANGES

Action

MAKING CHANGES

Clear goals (SMART)
Realistic plans
Support
+ve Reinforcement

Support
Reward (intrinsic)
Enjoyment
Motivation
Avoidance of risk

Preparer

PREPARING TO CHANGE

Minimize costs
Remove barriers
Reduce temptation to
fail (alternatives)
Encourage

Boredom
Circumstance changes
Lack of planning
High-risk situations
Lack of support
Lack of 'reward'

Pros/cons
Consider risks
Existing harm
Keeping a diary
Concerns

RELAPSING

Relapser

Pre-contemplator

Not interested in changing
'risky' lifestyle
**Health awareness
Check health
Identify risk factors
and knowledge
Provide information
Encourage/enable
exercise choice**

THINKING ABOUT CHANGE

Contemplator

Figure 3.5 Stages of change plus interventions, in the change model.[80 – 82]

provide the information about what was right or wrong about the original planning, in order to strengthen subsequent plans of action to recycle the relapser effectively on their next attempt.

Termination – stable 'safer' lifestyle, with no temptation to revert

This is regarded as a stable stage which is reached when the client has maintained the exercise behaviour for a period of over 5 years. The client is absolutely certain that they are able to maintain the behaviour despite any temptations there may be to revert back to the inactive state.

Although this stage is called 'termination' (in the context of this text, termination of physical activity), it is not the end of the client's behavioural journey. This process continues for the rest of their life, whether they remain active or not. It is useful to think of termination as representing a long-term consistency in the physically active behaviour. Being physically active has become part of the client's lifestyle.

Chapter summary

Figure 3.5 incorporates the interventions which are required at each stage into the stages of change model shown in Figure 3.4. The stage and a description of the client's intentions are shown in the outer rings and the interventions are incorporated in the inner segment. By following the interventions in each segment, the client can be helped to move successfully through the process of change.

References

1. Oxford University Press (1991) *Oxford English Dictionary*, OUP, London.
2. Atkinson, R.L., Atkinson, R.C., Bem, D.J. *et al.* (1990) *Introduction to Psychology*, 10th edn, Harcourt, Brace and Jovanovich, Philadelphia.
3. Dishman, R.K. (1988) *Exercise Adherence: Its Impact on Public Health*, Human Kinetics, Champaign, IL.
4. Dishman, R.K. (ed.) (1994) *Advances in Exercise Adherence*, Human Kinetics, Champaign, Il.
5. Biddle, S. and Mutrie, N. (1991) *Psychology of Physical Activity and Exercise. A Health Related Perspective*, Springer Verlag, New York.
6. Pate, R.R., Pratt, M., Blair, S.H. *et al.* (1995) Physical activity and public health. A recommendation from the Centres of Disease Control and Prevention and the American College of Sports Medicine. *J. A. M. A.*, **273**, 402–407.
7. Biddle, S. (1993) Children, exercise and mental health. *Int. J. Sports Psych.*, **24**, 200–216.
8. HMSO (1992) *The Health of the Nation: A Strategy for Health in England*, HMSO, London.
9. Yaffe, M. (1981) Sport and mental health. *J. Biosoc. Sports*, Suppl. 7, 89–95.
10. Rowland, T.W. (1990) *Exercise and Children's Health*, Human Kinetics, Champaign, IL.
11. Morgan, W.P. and Goldston, S.E. (1987) *Exercise and Mental Health*, Harper and Row, London.
12. Byrne, A. and Byrne, D.G. (1993) The effect of exercise on depression, anxiety, and other mood states: a review. *J. Psychosom. Res.*, **37**(6), 565–574.
13. North, T.C., McCullagh, P. and Tran, Z.V. (1990) Effects of exercise on depression. In *Exercise and Sports Science Reviews*, vol. 18 (Pandolf, K.B. and Holloszy, J., eds), Williams and Wilkins, Baltimore, MD.
14. Thirlaway, K. and Benton, D. (1992) Participation in physical activity and cardiovascular fitness have different effects on mental health and mood. *J. Psychosom. Res.*, **36**(7), 657–665.
15. Martinsen, E.W. (1993) Therapeutic implications of exercise for clinically anxious and depressed patients. *Int. J. Sports Psych.*, **24**, 185–199.
16. Petruzello, S.J., Landers, D.M., Hatfield, B.D. *et al.* (1991) A meta-analysis on the anxiety reducing effects of acute and chronic exercise. *Sports Med.*, **11**(3), 143–182.
17. Maroukalis, E. and Zarvas, Y. (1993) Effects of aerobic exercise on mood of adult women. *Perc. Mot. Skills*, **72**, 1203–1209.
18. Ossip-Klein, D.J., Doyne, E.J., Bowman, E.D. *et al.* (1989) Effects of running and weight lifting on self concept in clinically depressed women. *J. Cons. Clin. Psych.*, **57**, 158–161.

19. Bandura, A. (1977) Self-efficacy: toward a unifying theory of behavioural change. *Psych. Rev.*, **84**, 191–215.
20. Bandura, A. (1986) *Social Foundations of Thoughts and Action: A Social Cognitive Theory*, Prentice-Hall, Englewood Cliffs, NJ.
21. Stein, P.N. and Motta, R.W. (1992) Effects of aerobic and non-aerobic exercise on depression and self-concept. *Perc. Mot. Skills*, **74**, 79–89.
22. Doyne, E.J., Ossip-Klein, D.J., Bowman, E.D. *et al.* (1987) Running versus weight lifting in the treatment of depression. *J. Cons. Clin. Psych.*, **55**, 748–754.
23. Bosscher, R.J. (1993) Running and mixed physical exercise with depressed psychiatric patients. *Int. J. Sports Psych.*, **24**, 170–184.
24. Brandon, J.E. and Loftin, J.M. (1991) Relationship of fitness to depression, state and trait anxiety, internal locus of control and self control. *Perc. Mot. Skills*, **73**, 563–568.
25. Martinsen, E.W., Mehus, A. and Sandvik, L. (1985) Effects of aerobic exercise on depression: a controlled study. *Br. Med. J.*, **29**, 109–115.
26. Abramson, L.Y., Seligman, M.E.P. and Teasdale, J.D. (1978) Learned helplessness in humans: critique and reformulation. *J. Abnormal. Psych.*, **87**, 49–74.
27. Seligman, M.E.P. (1975) *Helplessnes: On Depression, Development and Death*, W.H. Freeman, New York.
28. Petruzello, S.J., Landers, D.M. and Salazar, W. (1993) Exercise and anxiety reduction: examination of temperature change as an explanation for affective change. *J. Sports Ex. Psych.*, **13**, 63–75.
29. Crocker, P.R.E. and Grozelle, C. (1991) Reducing induced state anxiety: effects of acute aerobic exercise and autogenic relaxation. *J. Sports Med. Phys. Fit.*, **31**, 277–282.
30. Lion, L.S. (1978) Psychological effects of jogging: a preliminary study. *Perc. Mot. Skills*, **47**, 1215–1218.
31. Butki, B.D. and Rudolph, D.L. (1997) Do short bouts of exercise reduce anxiety? *Med. Sci. Sports Ex.*, (suppl.), **29**(5), S118.
32. Biddle, S. (1995) Exercise and psychosocial health. *Res. Quart. Ex. Sports*, **66**(4), 292–297.
33. McGowan, R.W. and Pierce, E.E. (1991) Mood alterations with a single bout of physical activity. *Perc. Mot. Skills*, **72**, 1203–1209.
34. Berger, B.G. and Owen, D.R. (1988) Stress reduction and mood enhancement in four exercise modes: swimming, body conditioning, hatha yoga and fencing. *Res. Quar. Ex. Sports*, **59**, 148–159.
35. Steptoe, A., Edwards, S., Moses, J. and Matthews, A. (1989) The effects of exercise training on mood and perceived coping ability in anxious adults from the general population. *J. Psychosom. Res.*, **33**, 537–547.
36. Cockerill, I.M., Nevill, A.M. and Byrne, N.C. (1992) Mood, mileage and the menstrual cycle. *Br. J. Sports Med.*, **26**(3), 145–150.
37. Moses, J., Steptoe, A., Matthews, A. and Edwards, S. (1989) The effects of exercise training on the mental well being in the normal population: a controlled trial. *J. Psychosom. Res.*, **33**, 47–61.
38. Weinberg, R., Jackson, A. and Kolodny, K. (1988) The relationship of massage and exercise to mood enhancement. *Sports Psych.*, **2**, 202–211.
39. Wankel, L.M. (1993) The importance of enjoyment to adherence and psychological benefits from physical activity. *Int. J. Sports Psych.*, **24**, 151–169.
40. Campbell, R.N. (1984) *The New Science: Self-Esteem Psychology*, University Press of America, Lantham, MD.

41. Fox, K. (1990) *The Physical Self-Perception Profile Manual*, Office for Health Promotion. Northern Illinois University, DeKalb, IL.
42. Gruber, J.J. (1986) Physical activity and self esteem development in children: a meta analysis. In *Effects of Physical Activity on Children* (Stull, G.A. and Eckert, H.M., eds), Human Kinetics and American Academy of Physical Education, Champaign, IL.
43. McCauley, E. (1994) Physical activity; psychosocial outcomes. In *Physical Activity, Fitness and Health* (Bouchand, C. et al., eds), Human Kinetics, Champaign, Il., pp. 551–568.
44. Sonstroem, R.J. (1984) Self-esteem and physical activity. *Ex. Sports Sci. Reviews*, **12**, 123–155.
45. Fox, K.R. and Corbin, C.B. (1989) The physical self perception profile: development and preliminary validation. *J. Sports Ex. Psych.*, **11**, 408–430.
46. Sonstroem, R.J. and Morgan, W.P. (1989) Exercise and self esteem: rationale and model. *Med. Sci. Sports Ex.*, **21**, 329–337.
47. Feltz, D.L. (1983) Gender differences in the causal elements of Bandura's theory of self-efficacy on a high avoidance motor task. Paper presented at the North American Society for the Psychology of Sport and Physical Activity Conference, East Lansing. Mich.
48. Carron, A.V. (1984) *Motivation: Implications for Coaching and Teaching*, Sports Dynamics, London.
49. Health Education Authority (1995) *Becoming More Active: A Guide for Health Professionals*, HEA, London.
50. Sallis, J.F., Hovell, M.F. and Hofstetter, C.R. et al. (1989) A multivariate study of determinants of vigorous exercise in a community sample. *Prev. Med.*, **18**, 20–34.
51. Corbin, C.B. (1984) Self confidence of females in sport and physical activity. *Clin. Sports Med.*, **3**, 895–908.
52. Biddle, S. (1990) Keeping body and soul together: psychobiologic issues in exercise and health promotion. In *Proceedings of the Student Conference*, (Mercer, T., ed.), British Association of Sports Sciences, Leeds.
53. de Coverley Veale, D.M.W. (1987) Exercise dependence. *Br. J. Addiction*, **82**, 735–740.
54. Sheehan, G. (1983) The best therapy. *Phys. Sportsmed.* **11**, 43.
55. Morgan, W.P. (1979) Negative addiction in runners. *Phys. Sports Med.*, **7**, 57–70.
56. Morgan, W.P. and O'Connor, P.J. (1988) Exercise and mental health. In *Exercise Adherence; Its Impact on Public Health* (Dishman, R.K., ed.), Human Kinetics, Champaign, IL.
57. Morgan, W.P. and O'Connor, P.J. (1989) Psychological effects of exercise and sports. In *Sports Medicine* (Ryan, and Allman, eds), Academic Press, New York, pp. 671–689.
58. Peele, S. (1981) *How Much is Too Much?*, Prentice Hall, Englewood Cliffs, NJ.
59. McSherry, T.A. (1984) The diagnostic Challenge of anorexia nervosa. *Am. Family Phys.*, **29**(2), 141–145.
60. American College of Sports Medicine (1980) *Guidelines for Exercise Testing and Exercise Prescription*, Lea and Febiger, Philadelphia.
61. Morgan, W.P., Brown, D.R., Raglin, J.S. et al. (1987) Psychological monitoring of overtraining and staleness. *Br. J. Sports Med.*, **21**, 107–114.
62. Sapolsky, R.M. (1994) *Why Zebras Don't Get Ulcers. A Guide to Stress Related Diseases and Coping*, W.H. Freeman, New York.

63. Pierce, E.F., Olson, K.G. and Dewey, W.L. (1993) Beta-endorphin response to endurance exercise: relationship to exercise dependence. *Perc. Mot. Skills*, **77**, 767–770.

64. Daniel, M., Martin, A.D. and Carter, J. (1992) Opiate receptor blockade by naltrexone and mood state after acute physical activity. *Br. J. Sports Med.*, **26**(2), 111–115.

65. Dunn, A.L. and Dishman, R.K. (1991) Exercise and the neurobiology of depression. *Ex. Sports Sci. Rev.*, **19**, 41–98.

66. Chaouloff, F. (1989) Physical exercise and brain monoamines: a review. *Acta Phys. Scand.*, **137**, 1–13.

67. Morgan, W.P. (1985) Affective benefence of vigorous physical activity. *Med. Sci. Sports Ex.*, **17**, 94–100.

68. Stephens, T. (1988) Physical activity and mental health in the United States and Canada: evidence from four population surveys. *Prev. Med.*, **17**, 35–47.

69. Sonstroem, R.J. (1988) Psychological models. In *Exercise Adherence: Its Impact on Public Health* (Dishman, R.K., ed.), Human Kinetics, Champaign, IL.

70. Fentem, R.H., Bassey, E.J. and Turnbull, N.B. (1988) *The New Case for Exercise*, HEA, London.

71. Kirkcaldy, B.D. and Shephard, R.J. (1990) Therapeutic implications of exercise. *Int. J. Sports Psych.*, **21**, 165–184.

72. Robison, J.I. and Rogers, M.A. (1994) Adherence to exercise programmes: recommendations. *Sports Med.*, **17**(1), 39–52.

73. Martin, J.E. and Dubbert, P.M. (1985) Adherence to exercise. *Ex. Sports Sci. Rev.*, **13**, 137–164.

74. Health Education Authority (1992) *Allied Dunbar National Fitness Survey*. Sports Council and HEA, London.

75. Storlie, J. and Jordan, H.A. (1984) *Behavioural Management of Obesity*, Life Enhancement Publications, Champaign, IL.

76. Becker, M.H. and Maiman, L.A. (1975) Sociobehavioural determinants of compliance with healthcare and medical care recommendations. *Med. Care*, **13**, 10–24.

77. Kenyon, G.S. (1968) Six scales for assessing attitude towards physical activity. *Res. Quart.*, **39**, 566–574.

78. Fishbein, M. and Ajzen, I. (1975) *Belief, Attitude, Intention and Behaviour: An Introduction to Theory and Research*, Addison-Wesley, New York.

79. Ajzen, I. (1988) *Attitudes, Personality and Behaviour*, Open University Press, Buckingham.

80. Prochaska, J.O. (1979) *Systems of Psychotherapy: A Transtheoretical Analysis*, Dorsey Press, Homewood, IL.

81. Prochaska, J.O. and DiClemente, C.C. (1983) Stages and processes of self change of smoking: towards an integrative model of change. *J. Cons. Clin. Psych.*, **51**, 390–395.

82. Prochaska, J.C. and DiClemente, C.C. (1984) *The Transtheoretical Approach: Crossing Traditional Boundaries of Therapy*, Brooks/Cole, Pacific Grove, CA.

4
The science of aerobic exercise

> A brief history
> The science
> References

A brief history

This chapter provides a basic understanding of muscle energy metabolism, cardiorespiratory responses and adaptations to exercise. Before describing some of the fundamental physiology behind aerobic exercise training, however, it is felt that the reader should have an appreciation of how the science of aerobic exercise has been developed and how it has become such a popularly promoted cultural behaviour in Western society. The marathon is one of the most visible examples of the human body's ability to use oxygen for aerobically powering the muscles. The key requirement in performing aerobic acitivity is the ability to select the correct pace/intensity, where there is an optimum mixture of oxygen, fat and carbohydrate. The ancient Greek messenger, Pheidippides, extolled the virtues of pace selection and physical aerobic prowess, when in 490 BC he ran a 300 mile round-trip in 4 days to get a message to the Spartans to help the Athenians in their battle against the Persians. The message was, however, unsuccessful in persuading the Spartans to join the battle at Marathon, but the Athenians were still victorious over the Persians. Pheidippides then had to run 22 miles to Athens to announce the victory and inform the Athenians not to surrender to the Persian fleet.

In more recent history, Roger Bannister, as a young medical student, described a clear understanding of the role of oxygen, aerobic metabolism and pace/intensity in his scientific approach to breaking the four-minute mile, as quoted in his 1955 autobiography:[1]

The oxygen consumption of an athlete rises steeply as his speed increases. The miler is limited by lack of oxygen, and in order to keep his oxygen requirement to a minimum, would need to run at the slowest average speed to achieve his

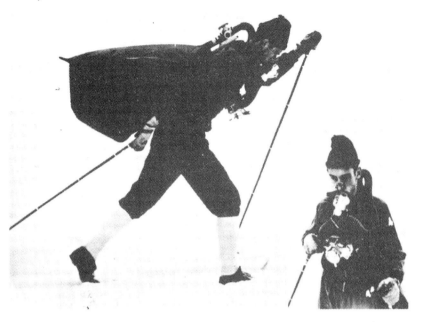

Figure 4.1 A Douglas bag experiment during cross-country skiing. (From Åstrand and Rodahl,[11] by courtesy of P.-O. Åstrand.)

target of a four-minute mile – the ideal would be four even laps of sixty seconds each.

Up to the 1950s

From the early part of the 1900s the study of the exchange of oxygen via the lungs, vital for muscle energy during exercise, has intrigued many scientists. The development of respiratory (breathing) analysis equipment (measuring the exchange of air between the lungs and the environment) quickly found its use in measuring exercise responses. One of the most notable pieces of equipment developed was the Douglas bag, where expired air was collected into a sealed bag and then analysed to see how much oxygen the body had used and how much carbon dioxide (CO_2) was produced (Figure 4.1). One Oxford lecturer from the 1940s and 1950s recalls seeing science students running around the college grounds with big bags on their backs connected via a tube to their mouth. They then quickly returned to the lab to analyse the content of oxygen and CO_2 that had been breathed into the bag (Figure 4.2a,b). Contents of the bag were fed through three different analysers – one for oxygen, one for CO_2 and one to measure the total volume of air which was collected over a set exercise period. From these three measures it is possible to determine how much oxygen is used during a particular activity.

Some laboratories still use this system because the technology is inexpensive, very reliable and it provides a valuable learning opportunity

(a)

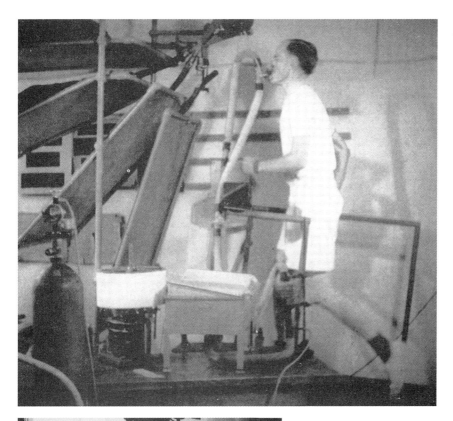

(b)

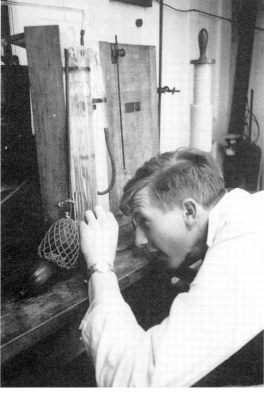

Figure 4.2 (a) Roger Bannister in 1951 as a young medical student carrying out treadmill experiments using the Douglas bag method; (b) analysis of the results with oxygen and carbon dioxide analysers. (Reprinted with permission of Hulton Getty Picture Library, London.)

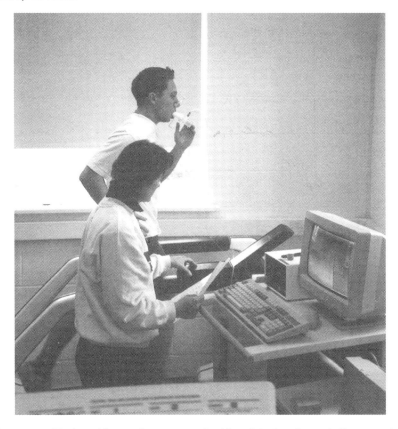

Figure 4.3 Testing with a modern computerized breath-by-breath metabolic cart analysis system at Keele University, UK.

for sports science and medical students to appreciate clearly the full analysis process. The running treadmill and exercise cycle ergometer proliferated alongside the Douglas bag procedure, which still today allows studies to be performed indoors, and also in sealed chambers where heat, humidity and pressure can be altered to measure responses to different environments. The time required to analyse expired air has now been greatly shortened with new computer technology and microanalysers, where immediate results of oxygen consumption and CO_2 production are given on a breath-by-breath basis (Figure 4.3). When the exercise test is complete, there is an immediate production of results.

The 1950s and 1960s

In the 1950s the Scandinavians led the way with their research into the physiology of respiration during exercise and also measuring respiration during manual labour in the workplace. The popular acknowledgement of the science of aerobic exercise climbed to new heights of public awareness with the pioneering work in the 1960s by Dr Ken Cooper. He coined the popularly known term 'aerobics', which today is often associated with exercise to music but includes any rhythmical activity that engages large muscle groups sustained for periods longer than 5 minutes.

The 1980s onwards

The wave of popularity of exercise to music 'aerobics' gained its greatest momentum in the early 1980s and created an almost overnight commercial success for a simple white shoe that carried a small embroidered Union Jack flag. The shoe was called 'Reebok' and its manufacturer continued to provide products for the aerobic exercise market with an activity called 'Step Reebok' (now simply called 'step' or 'step aerobics') and more recently the production of low-impact exercise walking machines. What will be next? Dr Cooper has developed a whole research centre in Dallas, the Aerobics Institute, specifically devoted to studying the science of aerobic exercise and its applications to health, fitness and rehabilitation.

The late 1970s through to the 1980s also saw the increased popularity and expansion of a 'gym culture', where the traditional multi-gym or universal gym weights equipment were separated into individual stations and designed much more ergonomically towards more effective muscular training. A company named Nautilus led the way with this sort of equipment by applying a concept known as variable resistance. The use of aerobic ergometers (cycles, rowers, treadmills, etc.) was, however, less important during these early periods of the gym culture and the gymnasiums therefore attracted individuals more interested in their muscles and shape rather than their health.

Into the mid and late 1980s more and more research on the benefits of aerobic exercise for health filtered through to the fitness industry and to the individual consumer. With the acknowledegement of aerobic exercise as the keystone to health-based activity, as outlined in Chapters 1–3, many of the companies who previously produced weights machines now concentrated their product development on 'high-tech' aerobic equipment. Aerobic exercise machines can be set for specific client needs, from elite training to cardiac rehabilitation. The merits of aerobic ergometers have more recently received attention with studies looking at which type of ergometers are the most effective in terms of energy (calorie) expenditure, and safety and effectiveness for rehabilitation patients.[2–6]

The science

A brief and basic understanding of the word 'aerobic'

There is a typical intuition among lay people that the word aerobic comes to mean the breathing of air and hence the more heavily one breathes the more aerobic the activity. This is almost the exact opposite to what is the true meaning of aerobic. The word 'aerobic' is short for aerobic metabolism, which is a process that occurs in the muscles and involves the microscopic exchange of oxygen in order to produce energy for muscle contraction. There is a link between this microscopic event and the breathing of the lungs, but as exercise intensity increases (Figure 4.7a, page 85), heavy breathing has been shown to be more a factor of the body getting rid of CO_2 than actually the taking in of more oxygen. In simple terms, the word 'aerobic' is more about what is happening in the muscles and not the lungs; during exercise the lungs are simply at the mercy of what the muscles are doing.

Cardiovascular/aerobic exercise in relation to other elements of exercise

In Chapter 1, exercise was defined as structured physical activity which focuses on the intent to improve one or a combination of all of the four basic elements of fitness (cardiovascular/aerobic endurance, muscular endurance, muscular strength and flexibility of muscles and joints).

The aim for improving any or all of the four components of fitness is wide ranging, from rehabilitation exercise and improving general health as a preventative measure, to enhancing specific sports performance. Some activities or sports rely specifically on one of the four elements of fitness. For example, competitive weight lifting is almost completely focused on muscular strength, whereas marathon running requires mainly cardiovascular aerobic endurance. Training programmes for some sports can become quite complex, because they entail all four elements of fitness to varying degrees, such as in team sports (soccer, basketball and hockey) or individual sports (tennis, skiing or the decathlon).

Responses and adaptations to exercise

The term 'responses' to exercise means those physiological parameters which become much more apparent and can either be felt or measured during activity, movement or exercise. These have been closely studied for centuries, even by the great philosophers and scientists (e.g. Leonardo da Vinci and Gallileo). Some of the typical responses being measured in today's exercise science laboratories include:

- breathing and ventilation (oxygen consumption and carbon dioxide production),
- blood profiles (red blood cell chemistry, fatty acids, cholesterol and lactic acid),
- muscle tissue chemistry,
- circulation (heart rate, blood pressure),
- psychological and social responses to exercise.

After a programme of exercise training, the amount of change in these responses can be measured, which is termed an 'adaptation'. The amount of adaptation of a physiological response at rest or during exercise is often correlated with a particular improvement in 'health' and/or 'fitness'. Changes in blood pressure, cholesterol, weight, heart strength and heart size would be considered 'health' adaptations. Changes in time and speed while performing a task (cycling, walking, running) or changes in lactic acid levels, breathing and oxygen consumption would be classified as 'fitness' adaptations. For purposes of health-related fitness, exercise scientists have studied the link between the health adaptations and the fitness adaptations and drawn conclusions on how daily physical tasks, general health, health risk reduction and quality of life are influenced.

As stated previously, a key element to health-related fitness is cardiovascular aerobic endurance, which is related to an individual's maximal aerobic capacity ($\dot{V}O_{2max}$).

$\dot{V}O_{2max}$ and its controlling factors

$\dot{V}O_{2max}$ is defined as the maximal volume of oxygen the body can take up and use, based upon three main physical aspects:

- the size and strength of the heart,
- the amount of blood a person has and the amount of oxygen the blood can carry,
- the amount of oxygen ($\dot{V}O_2$) the muscles can extract from the blood.

The ways in which $\dot{V}O_{2max}$ is measured or predicted will form an important part of Chapters 7 and 8. There are, however, a variety of occasions where exercise can be prescribed and performance can be evaluated without a $\dot{V}O_{2max}$ 'score'. The remaining sections of this chapter aim to illustrate the internal physical adaptations which occur with regular aerobic exercise. It is these changes, when regularly maintained, that confer the health benefits described in Chapter 2.

There are a number of factors which affect $\dot{V}O_{2max}$:

- *genetic make-up*, which can account for as much as 70% of a person's $\dot{V}O_{2max}$, which is dictated by heart size and strength and muscle fibre type,[7]
- *age*, where $\dot{V}O_{2max}$ naturally increases with growth up to about 20–25 years and then begins to decline at a rate of about 1% per year,[8]
- *gender*, where females on average have 15–30% lower aerobic capacities than males of a similar age and training status,[9]
- *the amount and intensity of exercise or activity regularly performed*, which can alter $\dot{V}O_{2max}$ usually by 10–20%; in some cases of very sedentary individuals or following long-term bed rest, it has been increased by 100%.[10]

Other factors which can affect $\dot{V}O_{2max}$ include: the type of activity (mode) performed, the number of large muscle groups being used, an individual's state of physical health and environmental factors including altitude and temperature (Figure 4.4).[11]

To date, genetic make-up and age are unchangeable factors, so the only controllable factor which can truly alter $\dot{V}O_{2max}$ is the amount of exercise and activity one performs.

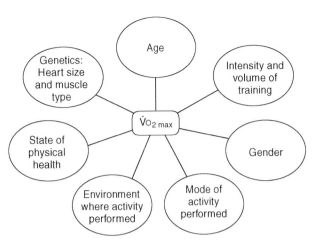

Figure 4.4 Factors which affect $\dot{V}O_{2max}$.

Means of expressing $\dot{V}O_{2max}$

$\dot{V}O_{2max}$ is usually expressed in one of two ways:

- in absolute terms as litres per minute (litres. min^{-1} or l. min^{-1}),
- relative to a person's body mass as millilitres per kilogram per minute ($ml. kg^{-1}. min^{-1}$).

In activities where body weight is supported, as on a stationary exercise cycle, then body weight plays a negligible part of the resistance and $\dot{V}O_{2max}$ can be expressed in absolute terms (litres. min^{-1}). With activities where the body weight is not supported by an external source, as in walking, running, climbing stairs or riding a bike up a hill, then $\dot{V}O_{2max}$ must be expressed in relation to body weight ($ml. kg^{-1}. min^{-1}$).

It is important to be able to convert $\dot{V}O_{2max}$ into either absolute or relative terms for two important reasons:

1. To fairly standardize the level of fitness between individuals with different body weights while performing the same weight-bearing activity (e.g. running).
2. To determine whether changes in health and fitness performance are a result of improved heart and muscle function, or weight loss or gain (or a combination of the two).

To further explain reason 1, a larger individual will most likely have a bigger heart, more blood and more muscle mass and thus a larger absolute $\dot{V}O_{2max}$. A key question for reasons of health and fitness is: Is this larger absolute $\dot{V}O_{2max}$ proportionally suitable to total body weight? With this question in mind it is important to be able to convert $\dot{V}O_{2max}$ into relative terms ($ml. kg^{-1}. min^{-1}$). A comparison can be made with an Austin Mini and a large truck both travelling on the motorway. Each engine can produce a maximum speed of 80 mph but the absolute power of the truck is probably 10 times that of the Mini. The ratio of engine power to car body weight is higher in the Mini, as seen by what happens when the two vehicles encounter the same hill; the truck loses power more quickly and climbs the hill more slowly than the Mini.

To further explain reason 2, a person who loses weight, without exercise training, will show an improved relative $\dot{V}O_{2max}$ (ml. kg^{-1}. min^{-1}) and may be able to perform exercise tasks to a higher level because they are lighter. If a person has trained regularly and lost weight, then both the improved heart and muscle fitness and the weight loss will have contributed to the improved exercise performance. To determine how much a person's improved exercise capability results from a training effect on the heart and muscles, the assessment must either compare

- exercise performance in a non-weight-bearing activity, or
- in absolute terms (litres. min^{-1}) of $\dot{V}O_{2max}$.

Understanding the importance of absolute and relative $\dot{V}O_{2max}$

An example would be in comparing two men who both have similar training regimens and the same absolute $\dot{V}O_{2max}$ of 3.0 litres min^{-1}. Both men can perform on the stationary exercise cycle and rowing machine to the same level, where their body weight is completely supported. When however they use the treadmill, one man can only sustain a walking pace of 6.5 kilometres per hour (kph) and the other can jog/run at 10 kph. The slower man on the treadmill weighs 100 kg, but the faster man only weighs 68 kg. The difference in their running/walking performance is explained by their relative $\dot{V}O_{2max}$ differences of 30 and 40 ml. kg^{-1}. min^{-1}, respectively.

To convert from an *absolute* $\dot{V}O_{2max}$ in litres. min^{-1} to a *relative* $\dot{V}O_{2max}$ in ml. kg^{-1} min^{-1}, the following formula is required:

$$\dot{V}O_{2max} \text{ (ml. kg}^{-1}\text{. min}^{-1}) = \text{Absolute } \dot{V}O_{2max} \text{ (litres. min}^{-1})$$
$$\times 1000 \text{ ml l}^{-1} \div \text{ Body mass (kg)}$$

To convert from a *relative* $\dot{V}O_{2max}$ in ml. kg^{-1}. min^{-1} to an *absolute* $\dot{V}O_{2max}$ in litres. min^{-1}, the following formula is required:

$$\dot{V}O_{2max} \text{ absolute (litres. min}^{-1}) = \text{Relative } \dot{V}O_{2max} \text{ (ml. kg}^{-1}\text{. min}^{-1})$$
$$\times \text{ Body mass (kg)} \div 1000$$

In Chapter 8 there is a full conversion chart which performs these calculations very quickly (Table 8.4).

Controllable factors for improving $\dot{V}O_{2max}$

The three main modifiable physical factors which can change $\dot{V}O_{2max}$ are:

1. The ability and strength of the heart to pump out blood (and thus oxygen) to meet the demands of the exercising muscles.

2. The ability of the muscles to extract and utilize oxygen from the blood.
3. The volume of oxygen which the blood can carry.[10,12]

I. Increased heart strength

When healthy but sedentary individuals take up regular exercise, all three of the above factors can be increased, which results in increased aerobic fitness performance. The main factor is an improvement in the strength of the heart.[10,13] For post heart attack patients performing rehabilitation exercise, where the heart muscle is damaged, improvements in aerobic fitness mainly occur from the muscles being able to extract and use more oxygen.[14]

2. Increased muscle oxygen extraction

Improvements in the ability of muscles to extract and use more oxygen from the blood is a result of three main factors following a period (6–10 weeks) of regular exercise training.[15–17]

- an increased number of capillaries (microscopic blood vessels) surrounding the muscle fibres, which allows a greater surface area over which oxygen can diffuse into the muscles,
- an increase in myoglobin (receptors and carriers of oxygen in the muscle cells),
- an increased volume of mitochondria (the specialized parts of the muscle cell, where oxygen is combined with glucose, fat and protein to produce energy).

3. Increased oxygen-carrying capacity of blood

Improvements in the oxygen-carrying capacity of the blood are related to an increased number of red blood cells.[12] Some endurance athletes have been known to increase their red blood cell count by 'blood doping'. In this procedure, performance is enhanced by injecting more red blood cells into the bloods stream and this enables the body to carry more oxygen. The practice of blood doping has been deemed unethical and could be medically harmful.[8]

Aerobic and anaerobic energy production

The first assumption about exercise is that skeletal muscles (those which move the limbs) are voluntarily activated from our own desire to use or contract them. Muscle energy for contraction is created by increasing the rate of production of a chemical known as adenosine triphosphate (ATP). This is produced either *aerobically*, where oxygen is required in the chemical reaction, or *anaerobically*, where ATP can be created very quickly without oxygen.

Aerobic production of ATP occurs, as stated above, in special parts of the cell called the mitochondria and involves the interaction of oxygen with the breakdown of a glucose-linked chemical, called pyruvate, and fat and protein. Because there is a limit to how much oxygen can be taken up by the mitochondria, aerobic production of ATP is slower than anaerobic production. Steady-state long-lasting activities, such as brisk walking, jogging and cycling, rely mainly on the aerobic production of ATP, which comes from a steady burning of fat as a fuel. As the intensity of activity is raised further and further, there is a point where the speed of ATP production cannot be met by the aerobic system and literally requires a boost from the anaerobic system. As one progresses towards this point the muscles have to rely less on fat as an energy source and more and more on carbohydrates (glucose and stored glycogen), which means the activity may not be sustainable. The optimal utilization of fat metabolism is linked to many health benefits of activity (i.e. reduced cholesterol and insulin resistance), which underpins the concept of longer, more frequent but lower intensity activity, as advocated in Chapters 1 and 2.

Figures 4.3 and 4.4 illustrate the link between the flow of oxygen and CO_2 to and from the muscle cell with the interplay of aerobic and anaerobic metabolism in creating ATP for muscle energy.

When *anaerobic production of ATP* is required, it produces a by-product known as lactic acid. If so much lactic acid is produced that it cannot be controlled or 'buffered' within the muscle cell, it spills into the blood stream. In order for the blood to perform its functions, there must be a good control or 'buffering' of any raised level of acidity. The blood has its own natural buffering system that reduces lactic acid, but with a chemical reaction that creates extra amounts of CO_2 in the blood. This excess CO_2 carried to the lungs needs to be literally 'blown out', which in theory[19] is a main contributor to a noticeable increase in the rate of breathing; the person starts to get a feeling of 'running out of puff'. At the same time, when lactic acid is accumulating and spilling out of the muscle into the blood stream there is a corresponding increase in muscle acidity, which interferes with the ability of the muscles to contract, and some pain or 'burn' can be felt. When this point of noticeable fatigue in the muscles occurs, either the intensity of the activity needs to be lowered or at more severe levels the activity must be stopped.

The concept of lactic acid accumulation in the blood was studied many years ago, in 1936,[20] and only a year later[21] it was established that the best way to help remove the lactic acid and recover more quickly from its effects was with light exercise; hence the idea of the post-exercise 'cool down' is nothing new.

It is the microscopic responses that occur in the muscles during exercise, which *drive* the more noticeable responses we can actually feel, including: breathing rate, heart rate, and degrees of pain or feelings of perceived exertion. Effective exercise prescriptions are based upon an understanding of these responses. It must, however, be appreciated that lactic acid is not the only contributor to heavier breathing; many other

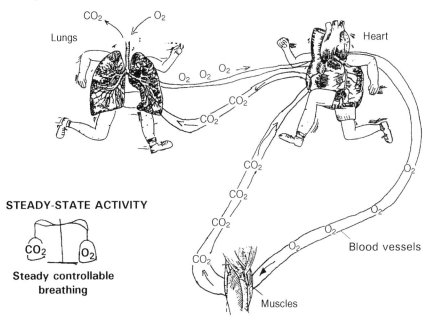

mechanical, chemical and pressure receptors located in the muscles, joints and blood vessels also send messages back to the brain which in turn contribute to driving the breathing mechanism. Figures 4.5 and 4.6 (and accompanying sketches) illustrate the pathways of oxygen and CO_2 circulation and the basic biochemistry of aerobic and anaerobic ATP production.

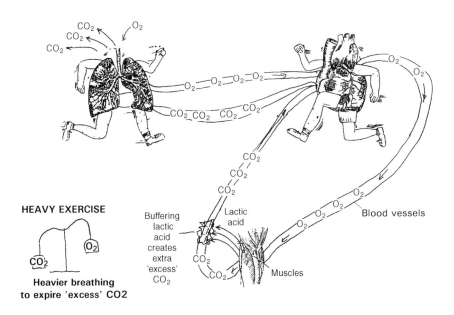

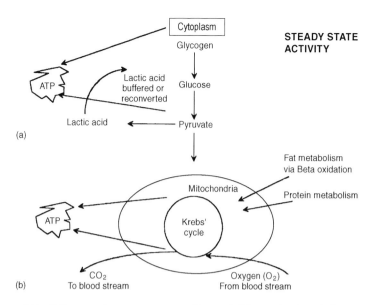

Figure 4.5 Pathways of oxygen consumption and CO_2 production during steady-state activity: (a) anaerobic metabolism; (b) aerobic metabolism. During steady-state exercise the breakdown of glucose to pyruvate to lactic acid is at a rate where any lactic acid produced is either buffered or reconverted into glycogen and glucose within the muscle cell. A majority of the production of ATP is met by the aerobic metabolism in the mitochondria, where oxygen combines with the carbon part of the broken-down pyruvate, fat or protein, which thus produces CO_2. The CO_2 is carried back to the lungs via the blood to be expired; breathing rate is raised during steady exercise but is controllable.

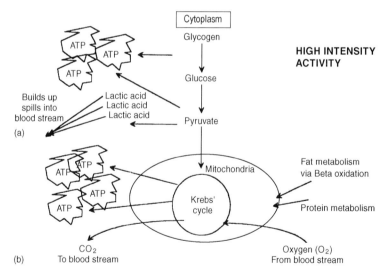

Figure 4.6 Pathways of oxygen consumption and CO_2 production during high-intensity activity: (a) anaerobic metabolism; (b) aerobic metabolism. During higher intensity exercise there is a much increased rate at which ATP energy needs to be produced and a boost is required by the anaerobic system to meet this demand; the aerobic system cannot meet the ATP production requirements fast enough. Lactic acid is therefore produced in greater quantities, accumulates and must be removed by the circulating blood to be carried away to be buffered and then reconverted into glycogen by other organs, including the liver and the heart muscle. (The number of ATP are not representative of true amounts of ATP produced. The diagrams are only to represent that high rates of ATP production are associated with the accumulation of lactic acid.)

Breathing responses and adaptations to exercise training

Breathing rate (ventilation rate) is probably the most noticeable response a person feels while exercising. As exercise intensity is increased, typical comments from the participant may include 'I'm feeling puffed' or 'I need to catch my breath'. From the authors' experience in carrying out thousands of post training fitness assessments over 9 years, clients have often commented that their lung capacity has improved because they now get 'less out of puff' during physical activities. Unfortunately there is little change in lung capacity or peak expiratory flow in reasonably healthy individuals when it is remeasured after a period of training,[11] which bemuses clients. A simple explanation, which can be offered to clients is:

As you get fitter, your heart, blood and muscles become more effective at delivering and utilizing oxygen; less CO_2 is produced and the response signals from the muscles and joints are dampened. This means your lungs do not have to work so hard at the same exercise level compared to when you were less fit. There is no actual change to the lungs – they are simply a filter for air, at the mercy of what your heart and muscles demand.

A more scientific understanding of changes in breathing from exercise training is illustrated in the graphical representations in Figure 4.7(a–d). In Figure 4.7(a), breathing rate (ventilation rate denoted as VE) increases in a straight line (linearly), with increased levels of exercise intensity, up to a point where breathing then becomes much more rapid, shown by the steep curve. At rest, a person breathes in and out (VE) about 6 litres of air per minute (litres.min^{-1}). Maximal VE during exercise can rise from 100 to 150 litres.min^{-1}, with extreme cases of elite endurance athletes reaching 200 litres.min^{-1}.[23] After a period of training (6–10 weeks), a higher intensity of exercise can be performed, before the steep increase in breathing rate occurs. The exercise intensity at the beginning of the exercise training programme, which initially caused rapid breathing, is now at a level where the breathing response is still linear (steady state). The point which the steep rise begins has been called the 'ventilatory threshold' and has been shown to correspond to either the 'anaerobic threshold' or point of onset of blood lactate accumulation (OBLA).[24,25] With training, this occurs at a higher percentage of a person's VO_{2max}. In healthy but more sedentary people, the anaerobic threshold occurs at 55–65% of VO_{2max}, in regularly trained individuals 65–75% VO_{2max}, while elite endurance athletes can sustain long-term exercise at up to 90% of their VO_{2max}.[11,22] This is discussed further in Chapters 5, 8 and 9.

In Figure 4.7(b), oxygen uptake (VO_{2max}) increases linearly with increased levels of exercise intensity and then reaches a maximum. At rest a person uses about 0.2–0.3 litres of oxygen per minute, but maximal oxygen uptake (VO_{2max}) or maximal aerobic capacity varies greatly, as stated earlier. For the cardiac or lung diseased patient, VO_{2max} may be as little as 1.5 litres.min^{-1},[26] which means that a steady walk may tax more than 80% of their whole aerobic capacity and causing breathing

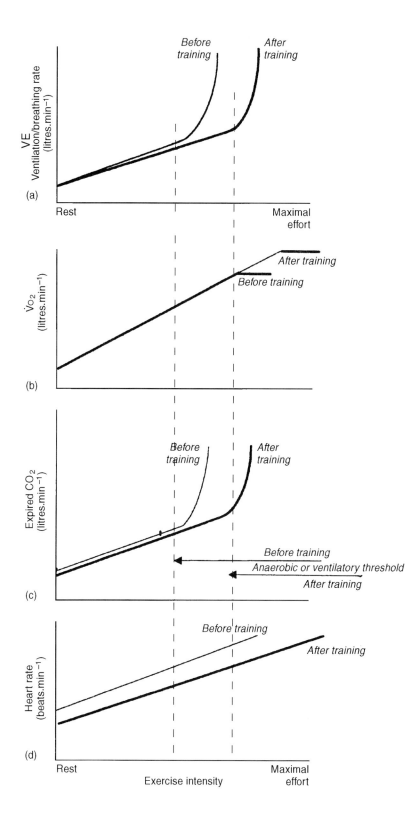

Figure 4.7 Cardiorespiratory changes after 6–10 weeks of training in a previously sedentary person. After training there is an increased $\dot{V}O_{2max}$ and the 'anaerobic or ventilatory threshold' occurs at a higher work rate and higher percentage of $\dot{V}O_{2max}$. (Adapted from Åstrand and Rodahl[11] and McArdle et al.[22])

85

rate to move to the curved part of the response in Figure 4.7(a). At the opposite end of the scale, an elite marathon runner, competitive cyclist or cross-country ski-racer may have an aerobic capacity between 4.5 and 6 litres min^{-1}.[11,27] At 80% of the elite endurance athlete's aerobic capacity, they have not yet reached the very steep part of the curve in Figure 4.7(a) and are able to sustain exercise equivalent to a running pace of 5 minutes per mile. Most healthy sedentary people will have a $\dot{V}O_{2max}$ in the range of 2–2.8 litres min^{-1} and the average person who regular exercises from 2.5 to 3.8 litres min^{-1}.[11]

At the beginning of the chapter it was outlined that a main contributing factor to $\dot{V}O_{2max}$ was genetics, with other key factors being the amount of regular training performed, age, gender and state of physical health. After a period of training, not only does $\dot{V}O_{2max}$ increase, but exercise can be performed at a higher percentage of this maximum before the onset of heavier breathing and/or the 'anaerobic/lactate threshold'.

In Figure 4.7(c), it can be seen that CO_2 production follows an almost parallel path with that of total ventilation shown in Figure 4.7(a). This shows that breathing rate is more related to expiring CO_2 than inspiring oxygen and that the lungs provide more than enough oxygen for the body during exercise.[11,22] Very similar to the ventilation response in Figure 4.7(a), after a period of exercise training, there is a shift to the right in the curve where more rapid breathing occurs at a higher intensity.

The information above gives a simplified version of factors which affect breathing during exercise. As noted earlier, there are many other factors which can be added to the complex process of triggering off increased breathing rate: strong emotional states and activation of stretch receptors in the joints and muscle tendons. The lungs even respond, prior to commencing joint movements of exercise, to hormonal and chemical changes in the blood that have been triggered by the 'thought' of exercising.

In Figure 4.8 is shown an actual print-out from a breath-by-breath analysis of an incremental exercise cycle ergometer test to determine $\dot{V}O_{2max}$. The print-out clearly shows that *during the submaximal stages* of the test, total ventilation (VE), oxygen consumption ($\dot{V}O_{2max}$) and carbon dioxide ($\dot{V}CO_{2max}$) all increased proportionally, where breathing response or ventilation (VE) were equally balanced between the demand for oxygen by the muscles and the CO_2 produced by the muscles. Between the dotted line region, VE and CO_2 begin to increase disproportionately to O_2 with increasing exercise intensity.

Nearer to *maximal levels of exercise* the increase in oxygen consumption ($\dot{V}O_{2max}$) plateaus but CO_2 continues to increase more steeply. This demonstrates the strong link between breathing rate and CO_2 production; it is not the lack of oxygen in the lungs that causes heavy breathing but a result of the higher content of CO_2 during higher intensities of exercise.

The lowered heart rate (pulse rate) following regular exercise training

After a period of training, many of the physiological adaptations described earlier are manifested in a decreased heart rate at rest and at

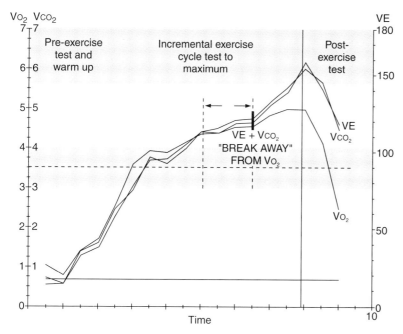

Figure 4.8 Breath-by-breath analysis of an incremental exercise cycle ergometer test to determine $\dot{V}_{O_{2max}}$. 'Break away' the intensity of activity where VE and $\dot{V}_{CO_2}$ increase at a greater rate than $\dot{V}_{O_2}$. VE = ventilation, $\dot{V}_{CO_2}$ = carbon dioxide production, $\dot{V}_{O_2}$ = oxygen consumption.

any given submaximal exercise intensity (Figure 4.7d). The electrical feedback system and nerve impulse control of the heart are related to four main training adaptations which were described earlier: (a) a stronger heart, (b) more blood vessels around the muscles, (c) better oxygen extraction by the muscles, and (d) more oxygen in the blood.

(a) From a stronger heart

It was stated earlier[10,13] that the heart muscle in healthy individuals becomes stronger following a period of training. The stronger heart pumps out a greater volume of blood (and thus oxygen) with each beat (known as the stroke volume). This means it does not have to beat so many times to get out the same volume of blood as compared to when it was less fit. At any given heart rate, then, there is a greater cardiac output. Cardiac output is the volume of blood pumped out each minute and is the product of heart rate × stroke volume. An increased cardiac output is a main feature of an increased $\dot{V}_{O_{2max}}$.[13]

(b) From more blood vessels (capillaries) around the muscles

Training, also stated earlier, increases the number of small blood vessels (capillaries) which feed the muscles, allowing for a greater volume of oxygen to pass through the muscle. This, in turn, reduces the number of times the heart has to beat in order to deliver a given amount of oxygen as compared to the blood flow of an untrained person.

(c) From improved oxygen extraction by the muscles

Another adaptation, following training, which reduces the number of times the heart has to beat for a given exercise intensity, is an improved ability of the muscles to extract oxygen from the blood. This is related to the increased volume of the mitochondria (oxygen processing unit and energy 'powerhouse' of the muscle) and myoglobin (oxygen receptors and carriers) inside the muscle cell. Again for a given volume of blood, more oxygen is taken from the muscle and therefore, for a given oxygen demand, less blood and fewer heart beats are required.

(d) From more oxygen in the blood

Finally, exercise training increases the oxygen-carrying capacity of the blood due to an increased production of red blood cells. There is a greater amount of oxygen per volume of blood and again the heart does not have to beat as many times to deliver the same volume of oxygen to the muscles.

Changes in the nervous/electrical control over heart rate

The turnover of oxygen or oxygen status in the muscle cells is detected by the nervous system and fed back to the central nervous system in the brain and brain stem. Both hormones and electrical signals are then released to either speed up or slow down the heart in relation to the oxygen demand of the muscles. With training, the oxygen delivery and muscle utilization capacity are enhanced, and the nervous system thus reduces its 'firing' rate on the heart both from a greater 'stroke volume' of the heart and a greater peripheral extraction and usage of oxygen by the muscles. Because training has no effect on increasing maximal heart rate,[23] the increased 'stroke volume' is completely responsible for the greater cardiac output which contributes to a greater VO_{2max}. It is important to understand that this is a very simplified description of heart rate control and that there are other factors which may also influence heart rate, including temperature, hormones and chemical responses, psychological state, and mechanical receptors in the blood vessels, lung muscles and skeletal muscles.

References

1. Bannister, R. (1955) *First Four Minutes*, Putnam Books, London.
2. Zeni, A.I., Hoffman, M.D. and Clifford, P.S. (1996) Energy expenditure with indoor exercise machines. *J. Am. Med. Assoc.*, **275**(18), 1424–1427.
3. Zeni, A.I., Hoffman, M.D. and Clifford, P.S. (1996) Relationships among heart rate, lactate concentration and perceived effort for different types of rhythmic exercise in women. *Arch. Phys. Med. Rehabil.*, **77**, 237–241.

4. Fulcher, K., Moore, J. and Evetts, S. (1997) A comparison of the physiological demands of exercising on selected home training devices. *J. Sports Sci.*, **15**(1), 50.

5. Urhauesen, A., Speildenner, J., Gabriel, H., Schwarz, L., Schwarz, M. and Kinderman, W. (1994) Cardiocirculatory and metabolic strain during rowing ergometry in coronary patients. *Clin. Cardiol.*, **17**, 652–656.

6. Buckley, J., Davis, J. and Simpson, T. (1997) Oxygen uptake during rowing ergometer and treadmill exercise 2 to 6 weeks post-myocardial infarction. Proceedings of the European Society of Cardiology Conference on New Insights in Cardiac Rehabilitation, Dublin, May.

7. Bouchard, C. and Malina, R.M. (1983) Genetics of physical fitness and motor performance. *Exerc. Sports. Sci. Rev.*, **11**, 306.

8. Astrand, I., Astrand, P-O., Hallback, I. and Kilbom, A. (1973) Reduction in maximal oxygen uptake with age. *J. Appl. Physiol.*, **35**, 649.

9. Drinkwater, B. (1973) Physiological responses of women to exercise. In *Exercise and Sport Science Reviews*, Vol. 1. (Wilmore, J., ed.), Academic Press, New York.

10. Saltin, B., Blomqvist, B., Mitchell, J.H. *et al.* (1968) Response to submaximal and maximal exercise after bed rest and training. *Circulation*, **38** (Suppl. 7), 1–78.

11. Astrand, P-O. and Rodahl, K. (1986) *Textbook of Work Physiology: Physiological Bases of Exercise*, McGraw-Hill, New York.

12. Ray, C.A., Kureton, C.J. and Ouzts, H.G. (1990) Postural specificity of cardiovascular adaptations to exercise training. *J. Appl. Physiol.*, **69**, 2202–2208.

13. Saltin, B. and Rowell, L.B. (1980) Functional adaptations to physical activity and inactivity. *Fed. Proc.*, **39**, 1506–1513.

14. O'Connor, G.T., Burning, J.E., Yusuf, S. *et al.* (1989) An overview of randomised trials of rehabilitation with exercise after myocardial infarction. *Circulation*, **80**, 234–244.

15. Howald, H. (1982) Training induced morphological and functional changes in skeletal muscle. *Int J. Sports Med.*, **3**, 1.

16. Hudlicka, O. (1982) Growth of capillaries in skeletal muscle. *Circ. Res.*, **50**, 451.

17. Pattengale, P.K. and Holloszy, J.O. (1967) Augmentation of skeletal muscle myoglobin by programmes of treadmill running. *Am. J. Physiol.*, **213**, 783.

18. American College of Sports Medicine (1996) Position stand: the use of blood doping as an ergogenic aid. *Med. Sci. Sports. Exerc.*, **28**(3), i–viii.

19. Loats, C.E.R. and Rhodes, E.C. (1993) Relationship between the lactate and the ventilatory threshold during prolonged exercise. *Sports Med.*, **15**(2), 104–115.

20. Bang, O. (1936) The lactate content of the blood during and after muscular exercise in man. *Scand. Arch. Physiol.*, **74**(Suppl. 10), 51.

21. Newman, E.V., Dill, D.B., Edwards, H.T. and Webster, F.A. (1937) The rate of lactic acid removal in exercise. *Am. J. Physiol.*, **118**, 457.

22. McArdle, W.D., Katch, F.I. and Katch, V.L. (1981) *Exercise Physiology: Energy, Nutrition and Human Performance*, Lea and Febiger, New York.

23. Saltin, B. and Astrand, P-O. (1967) Maximal oxygen uptake in athletes. *J. Appl. Physiol.*, **23**, 353.

24. Wasserman, K., Whipp, B.J., Koyal, S.N. and Beaver, W.L. (1973) Anaerobic threshold and respiratory gas exchange during exercise. *J. Appl. Physiol.*, **35**, 236–243.

25. Wasserman, K., Beaver, W.L. and Whipp, B.J. (1990) Gas exchange theory and the lactic acidosis (anaerobic) threshold. *Circulation*, **81** (Suppl. II), 14–30.

26. Pollock, M.L. and Schmidt, D.H. (1995) *Heart Disease and Rehabilitation*, Human Kinetics, Champaign, Il.

27. Newsolme, E. and Leech, T. (1985) *The Runner*. Walter L. Meager, Oxford.

5
The importance of understanding and acknowledging training status

Potential
Appreciating $\dot{V}O_{2max}$, only when considered alongside training status
References

It seems appropriate to begin writing this chapter on the day of the London Marathon. One cannot help but admire those tens of thousands of participants, ranging from the very elite to the charity fund-raisers wearing costumes. Most of the admiration is knowing one common factor to a large proportion of these participants – the time and effort they have put into their *training* over many miles and many months of preparation.

Training is something which is performed to different levels and is of different types. If a person does very little activity they are considered to be 'sedentary', whereas elite marathon runners are termed 'highly trained'. There are, however, many non-elite athletes who are also highly trained and possibly doing as much as some elite competitors do; but why are they not finishing in the top places of the marathon? It stems back to the facts outlined in Chapter 4 on the genetic influences on aerobic capacity. Those individuals born with large hearts and appropriate muscle fibres have a greater potential.

Potential

The word 'potential' is very important. A person can train with the most advanced techniques, but without the genetic potential may never be able to break the marathon time barrier that continues to be just out of their grasp. For some, this barrier is 4 hours, for others it is 3 hours and now, for the top athletes, that infamous 2-hour barrier.

In recollecting the discussions in Chapter 4, $\dot{V}O_{2max}$ is as much if not more a measure of an individual's potential as opposed to a measure of how much they train; unless of course they have had long bouts of bedrest or been chairbound or very sedentary. The importance of acknowledging training status is highlighted by the fact that since the 1930s the scores of $\dot{V}O_{2max}$ in elite endurance athletes have increased very little in comparison to the large increases in performance times.[1,2] The answer to this problem must then lie with the methods and volume of training used by today's athletes and their ability to sustain exercise at a higher percentage of their $\dot{V}O_{2max}$ ('potential') than in previous eras. The following example may be more helpful in relation to individuals performing health-related exercise.

Example

Two 45-year-old females of almost the same height and weight have volunteered to be subjects in a study, which is being carried out by the nearby university sports science department. After completing a pre-test health screening, they were both cleared to be tested on the treadmill, with full respiratory analysis, to determine $\dot{V}O_{2max}$.

Ms A. attained a $\dot{V}O_{2max}$ of 38 ml. kg^{-1}. min^{-1} and Ms B. one of 45 ml. kg^{-1}. min^{-1}. It was part of the study protocol for the ladies not to be told their $\dot{V}O_{2max}$ score until the end of the whole research project in 2 months time. The next day both ladies entered a 3-mile charity fun run/walk. Not knowing their fitness scores, they made a bet that whoever took longer to complete the 3 miles would have to give £5 to the charity. Ms A., who had the lower $\dot{V}O_{2max}$, actually won by over $1\frac{1}{2}$ minutes; how could this be?

Ms A. does not have a car and walks 2.5 miles to work and back each day, swims for half an hour 3 times per week during her lunch break and attends an aerobics class on Tuesday night and Saturday morning.

Ms B. is an executive accounting director in the City, her job entails a lot of driving and she often works a 12-hour day. As a result of her work, she claims to have little leisure time. The last time she did any regular training was at university, where she performed to a high standard as a member of the cross-country running team.

Ms A. can be categorized as having a 'training status' of 'regularly trained and highly active'. From the concepts discussed in Chapter 4 on 'anaerobic or ventilatory thresholds', her training status allows her to sustain activity at a level up to 75% of her $\dot{V}O_{2max}$. Her functional (steady-state) oxygen uptake is therefore:

$$75\% \ \dot{V}O_{2max} \ \text{of} \ 38 \ \text{ml. kg}^{-1}. \ \text{min}^{-1} = 28.5 \ \text{ml. kg}^{-1}. \ \text{min}^{-1}$$

or being able to sustain a jogging pace of 10:45 (min:sec) per mile via aerobic metabolism (see Chapter 8).

Ms B. is categorized as 'sedentary', as her daily routines have little continuous activity and she does not regularly participate in any structured exercise. She can therefore only sustain a level of activity up to 60% of her $\dot{V}O_{2max}$. Her functional oxygen uptake is actually lower than Ms. A.'s, which explains her poorer performance over the 3-mile run, shown by the following calculation:

$$60\% \ \dot{V}O_{2max} \text{ of } 45 \text{ ml. kg}^{-1}. \text{ min}^{-1} = 27 \text{ ml. kg}^{-1}. \text{ min}^{-1}$$

or being able to sustain a jogging pace of 11:15 (min:sec) per mile via aerobic metabolism.

Ms B.'s 'potential' to perform is, on the other hand, far greater than Ms A.'s. If she were to perform regular aerobic training, she could increase her $\dot{V}O_{2max}$ by 10–20% (see Chapter 4) and would also be able to work at a higher percentage of this as well. With regular training, Ms B.'s functional oxygen uptake could be calculated by adding at least 10% to her present $\dot{V}O_{2max}$ and then taking 75% of this new score:

$$45 \text{ ml. kg}^{-1}. \text{ min}^{-1} + 10\% = \text{approx. } 50 \text{ ml. kg}^{-1}. \text{ min}^{-1}$$

then

$$75\% \text{ of } 50 \text{ ml. kg}^{-1}. \text{ min}^{-1} = 37.5 \text{ ml. kg}^{-1}. \text{ min}^{-1}$$

Ms B.'s improved aerobic fitness would mean that her functional (steady-state) oxygen uptake could almost be 10 ml. kg^{-1}. min^{-1}. greater than Ms A.'s (37.5 − 28.5). This would be equivalent to adding more than 3 km per hour to Ms B.'s running speed (see Chapter 8). If, as discussed in Chapter 4, Ms B.'s age is then taken into account, where there is a decrease of 1% per year in her $\dot{V}O_{2max}$, it clearly shows why she was a member of the university cross-country team 25 years earlier. Her $\dot{V}O_{2max}$ at age 20 on these calculations would have been near 60 ml. kg^{-1}. min^{-1}, typical of high-level female endurance athletes.

Because Ms. A. is already well trained, her $\dot{V}O_{2max}$ cannot increase much more and even if she intensified her training schedule to enable her to work at best at 85% of her $\dot{V}O_{2max}$ (34 ml. kg^{-1}. min^{-1}), she would still not match Ms. B.'s performance capabilities attained from a moderate regular training programme.

Appreciating $\dot{V}O_{2max}$, only when considered alongside training status

The example given above of two similarly aged females highlights how exercise professionals must consider both the present capabilities and potential future goals and aims of each individual client. Obtaining a clear history of exercise training in the past 12 months and acknowledging any performance standards attained in the longer term history is a paramount component of any exercise consultation. The last chapter of this book is devoted to considering such matters along with the health and psychosocial profile of the client. It is somewhat disappointing to see that some of the fitness test procedures used within the health and fitness industry give ratings from poor to good on $\dot{V}O_{2max}$ alone, without consideration of a person's activity history and how sedentary or active a person is at present.

Figure 5.1 has been adapted from the research outlined in Chapter 4,[1–14] and illustrates the relationship between training status and the

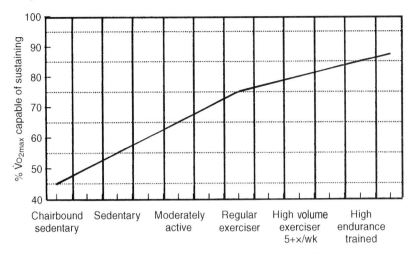

Figure 5.1 Training status and how it affects the percentage $\dot{V}O_{2max}$ which can be sustained. (An adaptation from research on respiratory and skeletal muscle biochemical processes with exercise training.[1-14])

Table 5.1 Training status and percentage $\dot{V}O_{2\ max}$ capability

Training status	% $\dot{V}O_{2\ max}$ capable of sustaining
Sedentary	55–65%
Moderate to regularly active or trained	65–75%
Highly trained	75–90%

percentage of a person's aerobic capacity that can be utilized during endurance activities.

Table 5.1 is a key component for the exercise prescription chapters to follow.

References

1. Astrand, P-O. (1956) Human physical factors with special reference to sex and age. *Physiol. Rev.*, **36**, 307.
2. Astrand, P-O. and Rodahl, K. (1986) *Textbook of Work Physiology: Physiological-Bases of Exercise*, McGraw-Hill, New York.
3. Saltin, B., Blomqvist, B., Mitchell, J.H. *et al.* (1968) Response to submaximal and maximal exercise after bed rest and training. *Circulation*, **38** (Suppl. 7), 1–78.
4. Saltin, B. and Rowell, L.B. (1980) Functional adaptations to physical activity and inactivity. *Fed. Proc.*, **39**, 1506–1513.
5. Howald, H. (1982) Training induced morphological and functional changes in skeletal muscle. *Int. J. Sports Med.*, **3**, 1.

6. Hudlicka, O. (1982) Growth of capillaries in skeletal muscle. *Circ. Res.*, **50**, 451.
7. Pattengale, P.K. and Holloszy, J.O. (1967) Augmentation of skeletal muscle myoglobin by programmes of treadmill running. *Am. J. Physiol.*, **213**, 783.
8. American College of Sports Medicine (1990) Position stand: the recommended quantity and quality of exercise for developing and maintaining cardiorespiratory and muscular fitness in healthy adults. *Med. Sci. Sports. Exerc.*, **22**(2), 265–274.
9. Loats, C.E.R. and Rhodes, E.C. (1993) Relationship between the lactate and the ventilatory threshold during prolonged exercise. *Sports Med.*, **15**(2), 104–115.
10. McArdle, W.D., Katch, F.I. and Katch, V.L. (1981) *Exercise Physiology: Energy, Nutrition and Human Performance*, Lea and Febiger, New York.
11. Saltin, B. and Astrand, P-O. (1967) Maximal oxygen uptake in athletes *J. Appl. Physiol.*, **23**, 353.
12. Wasserman, K., Whipp, B.J., Koyal, S.N. and Beaver, W.L. (1973) Anaerobic threshold and respiratory gas exchange during exercise. *J. Appl. Physiol.*, **35**, 236–243.
13. Wasserman, K., Beaver, W.L. and Whipp, B.J. (1990) Gas exchange theory and the lactic acidosis (anaerobic) threshold. *Circulation*, **81** (Suppl. II), 14–30.
14. Newsolme, E. and Leech, T. (1985) *The Runner*. Walter L. Meager, Oxford.

6

Monitoring exercise responses: heart rate, ratings of perceived exertion and blood pressure

Heart rate
Ratings of perceived exertion
Blood pressure
References

The next four chapters specifically focus on the measurement, evaluation and prescription of cardiovascular-based exercise. Heart rate and Borg's 15-point Rating of Perceived Exertion Scale (RPE)[1] are featured throughout these chapters as the key 'markers' for measuring and evaluating exercise status for practice/field-based work. Understanding blood pressure response during exercise is another means of ensuring that a safe and effective level of exercise is being performed, either during testing or programme monitoring. Without first establishing the rudiments of heart rate, RPE and blood pressure, the chapters to follow would be meaningless.

Heart rate

Heart rate is defined as the number of times the heart beats in 1 minute, which gives a clear idea of the strain upon or work required of the heart muscle at any given time. Each time the heart beats it creates a pulse or 'wave' of blood which flows from the heart, driving both systemic circulation (blood flow to peripheral tissues, organs and the brain) and pulmonary circulation (to the lungs). Heart rate response to exercise, as described in Chapter 4, is directly related to the oxygen demand of the muscles. The ease of being able to monitor heart rate and its direct relationship with oxygen usage (oxygen uptake or $\dot{V}O_2$) is the reason why heart rate has become probably the most commonly measured exercise response.

The pulse of the blood, created from the contraction of the heart's ventricles (lower chambers), can easily be felt (palpated) at various sites on the body including the carotid artery in the neck, the radial artery near the wrist and the femoral artery in the groin area. It is, however, difficult to palpate an individual's pulse during exercise in order to measure heart rate. Because of the movement, taking one's pulse accurately to monitor the effects of exercise, except during stationary exercise cycling, means that the individual will have to at least briefly stop and thus a true exercising heart rate is not obtained. To overcome the problem of palpating a pulse during exercise, various types of heart rate monitors have been devised. Some of these types of monitors will be briefly discussed before further discussing heart rate.

Instruments for measuring heart rate or pulse rate

It is important to have an appreciation of the types of monitor available and to acknowledge their limitations when used for measuring heart rate response during exercise.

Pulse monitors

These monitors typically employ a fingertip or earlobe probe and usually work on one of three principles: a light beam, an infrared reflector beam, or a pressure-sensitive switch. When the pulse of blood passes through the light or infrared beam or physically triggers the pressure-sensitive switch it is registered on the monitor as one beat. The time interval between each of these beats is then used in calculating the heart rate in beats per minute. Many monitors can be quite accurate, but only when the probe is kept very still. Stationary exercise cycling provides one of the few situations where the probe can be kept very still. Factors which often compromise measurement accuracy of probe-based monitors include:

- perspiration getting on the probe, with the residual salt creating a short lifespan of the probe,
- skin pigments interfering with light-based probes,
- irregular heart beats (arrhythmias),
- the probe being moved and creating false beats known as 'movement artefacts/noise'.

Ensuring that equipment is not faulty and is regularly checked, prevents anxiety in clients who think that the unusual response is possibly a physical problem with their heart or circulation (Figures 6.1 and 6.2).

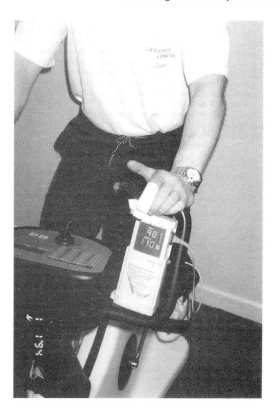

Figure 6.1 Heart rate measured by pulse oximeter in use during exercise cycling.

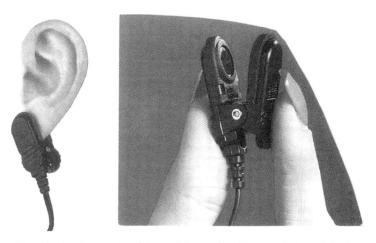

Figure 6.2 Heart rate monitored by earlobe probe. (By permission of Bodycare Ltd, Warwick, UK.)

Electrocardiograms

Electrocardiograms (ECGs) are the most accurate tool for measuring heart rate. From the ECG signal (Figure 6.3), which directly measures the electrical activity controlling the heart, heart rate is calculated by measuring the time interval between the spikes of the QRS wave. Some of the better monitors are able to make accurate heart rate calculations in spite of the presence of arrhythmias or unusual (ectopic) waveforms.

Exercise ECG systems are often very costly owing to the accuracy needed to assess cardiac patients during a treadmill stress test, where any artefacts/noise created by the movement of the leads, cables or electrodes on the skin are filtered. More basic systems (Figure 6.4) are designed to assume the body remains still and may only be useful for use with a stationary exercise cycle.

Even with some basic systems, special training is required to use an ECG, and the user needs to clearly show their confidence if they are using it on a client. The exercise professional must carefully consider their level of training, and the cost and practicalities of using an ECG, before making the decision to use this type of monitoring system.

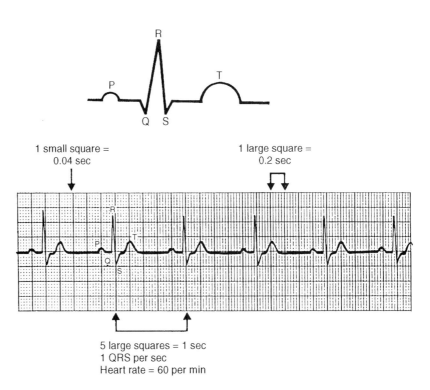

Figure 6.3 A basic ECG trace. P = electrical stimulation which leads to pumping of the atria (upper chambers); QRS = electrical stimulation of ventricles, where blood is pumped out to the lungs and to the head and rest of the body. T = repolarization (electrical resetting) of ventricles preparing the heart for another cycle of pumping. The time period between QRS waves = I pulse and when counted over I minute gives a pulse rate in beats per minute.

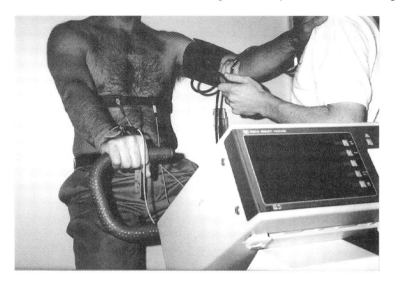

Figure 6.4 A three-lead ECG system for accurately monitoring heart rate during a cycle ergometer test.

Wireless chest strap personal heart rate monitors

These were first introduced in the early to mid-1980s and have revolutionized the ability for almost anyone to monitor their heart rate very accurately during practically any form of activity, including swimming (Figure 6.5). Within five minutes of putting the chest strap on most people will claim 'you forget that you even have it on'.

The chest strap has two electrodes, which work on the same principle as the ECG, by directly picking up the electrical impulses controlling the heart. On the strap is a radiotransmitter. The transmitter sends a signal of the spike in the ECG QRS wave to a receiver wrist watch, which calculates and displays heart rate in beats per minute. Some watches can record many hours of heart rate responses, which can then be downloaded to a computer for analysis. This system is widely used, from high-level athletes (cyclists, runners, rowers) to gym-based exercisers and cardiac rehabilitation patients.

For practicality and use by health-based exercise professionals, both for testing and training, the chest strap heart rate monitor is probably the most recommended device if heart rate is the only measure required. However, it too has its limitations, including:

- interference of the radio signal between the strap and the watch by other nearby electromagnetic appliances (e.g. electric motors, car alternators),
- the present technology is not able to correct for arrhythmias of the heart and may give false readings,
- the wire sutures which hold the sternum (breast bone) together in coronary bypass patients may interfere with the signal,

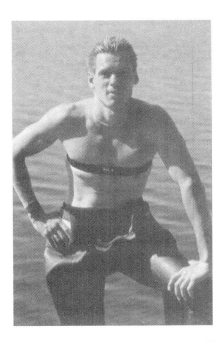

Figure 6.5 A wireless chest strap heart rate monitoring system. The two chest electrodes pick up the QRS wave and transmit the signal via radio waves to a wrist watch receiver, which calculates and converts the signals into a heart rate based on the time period between QRS waves. (By permission of Bodycare Products, Warwick, UK.)

- if two people wearing heart rate monitor chest straps stand too close together their radio signals may interfere with each other, but some newer systems may use different transmitter frequencies so that this does not occur.

Many of the modern aerobic exercise machines have built-in receivers that are compatible with most chest strap transmitters. Some machines can automatically adjust the resistance or pace from the target heart rate programmed into the machines' computer.

Hand grip sensors

These sensors work on a pressure-sensitive system which pick up the physical circulation pulse in the hands. Recent technology has developed much more accurate devices which have been fitted to some exercise machines including cycles and steppers. The sensors again assume that the heart has a normal rhythm pattern.

Heart rate response with exercise

The reasons why heart rate rises with with increasing levels of exercise intensity, and why after a period of regular training it slows down both at rest and at a given intensity of exercise, are addressed in Chapter 4.

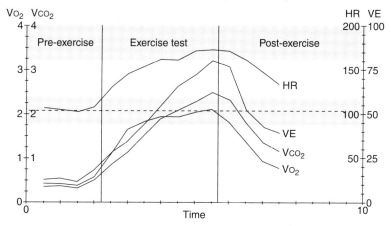

Figure 6.6 The relationship between oxygen consumption ($\dot{V}O_2$) and heart rate (HR) before, during and after an exercise test, from an actual printout of respiratory gas analysis and heart rate during exercise. Note how heart rate follows a parallel path to oxygen uptake, thus showing how heart rate provides a clear representation of energy demand through its direct relationship with oxygen consumption.

The overriding factor during exercise, which affects heart rate, is the need to deliver oxygen to the exercising muscles. During submaximal activity there is a direct linear relationship between oxygen consumption ($\dot{V}O_2$) and heart rate (HR).[2] This is the reason why the world of exercise science has paid so much attention to heart rate response as a means of externally (non-invasively) monitoring energy demand during exercise. Figure 6.6 clearly demonstrates such a relationship as shown during an exercise test where $\dot{V}O_2$ and HR follow almost a perfectly parallel path, before, during and following an exercise test.

Maximal heart rate (HR$_{max}$)

As the reader progresses through the next few chapters it will become evident that much of the general field-based exercise prescriptions and test protocols being used are based on the concept of maximal heart rate (HR$_{max}$). Such a concept has very close links with that of maximal oxygen uptake ($\dot{V}O_{2max}$), where it is used as a 'marker' of a person's maximal exercise capacity. It is of course much easier to measure HR$_{max}$ than $\dot{V}O_{2max}$, but similar to $\dot{V}O_{2max}$ it is often not practical, or safe, to push clients to high levels of intensity to actually determine HR$_{max}$. It is possible to estimate or predict HR$_{max}$, as noted in a separate section below. Furthermore, because there is a direct relationship between HR and $\dot{V}O_2$ and thus HR$_{max}$ and $\dot{V}O_{2max}$, HR and HR$_{max}$ have been widely used in many test protocols for estimating or predicting $\dot{V}O_{2max}$ which will be described in Chapter 8.

Age and maximal heart rate

The relationship between age and maximal heart rate has been researched for many decades, with major studies from Robinson in the

1930s[3] to Astrand in the 1950s[4] and Londeree in the 1980s.[5] It is now well established from these studies that, after the age of 10 years, maximal heart rate declines about 1 beat per minute (bpm) per year. During the period between ages 10 and 25 years this decline is probably due to the increasing size and strength of the heart and the corresponding development of the nervous system which controls the heart. After the age of 25, like all other tissues in the body, the slow ageing deterioration of the heart begins. It is interesting to note that after the age of 25 there is a 1% per year decline in potential $\dot{V}O_{2max}$ which coincides with the decline in maximal heart rate. These coinciding declines in HR_{max} and $\dot{V}O_{2max}$ would seem sensible alongside other close relationships between the size and strength of the heart (stroke volume and cardiac output) and $\dot{V}O_{2max}$, as noted in Chapter 4.

Acknowledging the decline in cardiac function with age again highlights the importance of maintaining regular activity throughout life. As noted in Chapter 2, being active and/or fitter enables one to cope better with the declining physical factors of ageing and the prevention of the premature onset of coronary heart disease.

Estimating HR$_{max}$

The general result from the studies noted in the above paragraphs is that on average, for both men and women, maximal heart rate can be estimated by the calculation of 220 minus age ($HR_{max} = 220 - $ age). Some caution with this calculation is advised, as 5–10% of people's HR_{max} can be as much as 20 bpm above or below this average level. Furthermore, this variability becomes more apparent with an increase in age;[5] therefore, this calculation is much more valid in younger than in older individuals. Chapter 7 will further look at this relationship between age and maximal heart rate and how it is applied in exercise programming.

With the potential variability in age predicted HR_{max} (Figure 6.7) or sometimes the inability to measure heart rate accurately, as noted earlier, what other simple field-based measures can be taken to monitor an individual's relative effort to ensure that effective and safe activity or training occurs? One answer is the use of ratings of perceived exertion (RPE).

Ratings of perceived exertion

A rating of perceived exertion is '. . . the act of detecting and interpreting sensations from the body during physical exertion'.[6] The use of Borg's RPE scale, in spite of its very simple 'cardboard' technology, has now become as much an accepted tool in sports and exercise science as that of heart rate. Its use ranges from exercise testing, monitoring and prescription,[7] to the training of elite athletes and the rehabilitation of cardiopulmonary patients.[8–10]

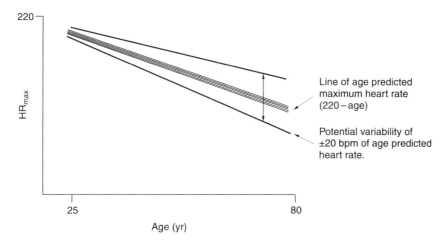

Figure 6.7 The variability in age-predicted maximal heart rate. The variability of prediction increases with age, up to 20 bpm either side of maximum predicted heart rate. (Adapted from Robinson,[3] Astrand *et al.*[4] and Londeree and Moeschberger[5].)

A brief background to RPE

Gunnar Borg, from Sweden, is credited with developing the now widely used rating scale of perceived exertion. Since its conception in the late 1950s it has evolved and been researched heavily by testing its relationship with numerous psychological and physiological responses, including pain, breathing rate, heart rate, oxygen consumption and lactic acid accumulation, in both healthy and clinical populations.[11]

The scale used in this text (Figure 6.8) is the modified 15-point scale first established in 1971, which is probably the most widely used RPE

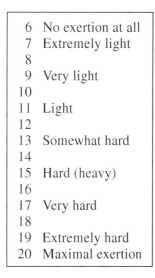

6	No exertion at all
7	Extremely light
8	
9	Very light
10	
11	Light
12	
13	Somewhat hard
14	
15	Hard (heavy)
16	
17	Very hard
18	
19	Extremely hard
20	Maximal exertion

Figure 6.8 Borg's 15-point RPE Scale. (By permission of Gunnar Borg[12].)

scale in sports and exercise science to date. One may wonder why it goes from 6 to 20 rather than 1 to 15. The reason for the 6 to 20 scale is because it was originally established for use with middle-aged men in order to predict exercise heart rate. If the RPE value is multiplied by 10, this would predict the heart rate at that intensity. For example, an RPE of 6, equating to sitting still (no exertion at all) represents a heart rate of 60, which is the average resting heart rate of a middle-aged man. At the other end of the scale, an RPE of 18–20 (maximal exertion), when multiplied by 10 (180–200) equates to the average maximal heart rate of a middle-aged man, remembering that maximal heart rate is estimated by 220 minus age, as noted earlier in this chapter.

Although research has now shown that the relationship between RPE and heart rate is not as strong as RPE with other physiological measures like breathing rate, oxygen consumption or lactic acid levels, the 6–20 scale has remained the accepted norm. Dishman,[13] a leading psychological adviser to the American College of Sports Medicine, has cited that RPE is more closely linked with relative oxygen consumption ($\dot{V}O_2$) than with relative heart rate.

Noble and Robertson,[6] who have worked closely with Borg, have written a comprehensive text on RPE, which is recommended for anyone wishing a more detailed understanding. The book, simply entitled *Perceived Exertion*, covers the extensive development of RPE and its use up to the late 1980s. Research since 1990 has proliferated, including:

- patient populations (CHD, lung disease),
- its validity when used with children,
- its use in a wide variety of activity modes,
- a variety of methods of application (estimated or produced exertion, and preferred exertion) which will be discussed later.

Mediators or factors influencing RPE

The general concept behind RPE is that it is a single, overall or integrated rating from numerous body response signals during exercise which converge on the brain's sensory cortex.[14] These sensations are filtered out by the brain which a person then perceives as a single rating, expressed verbally using the 15-point RPE scale. Figure 6.9 illustrates the flow of sensations which lead to the giving of an RPE.

Ensuring the effective use of RPE

At first glance one might look at an RPE scale and ask: How can a subjective rating scale be a valid tool for measuring exercise intensity? It is probably the defence against such a question that has led to the mountain of research which has piled up since the late 1950s when Gunnar Borg conceptualized his rating scale of perceived exertion.

If a measurement tool is used incorrectly, then of course it will be doomed to invalidity. Often the downfall of much exercise science research is the failure to apply it easily into an everyday setting. Such

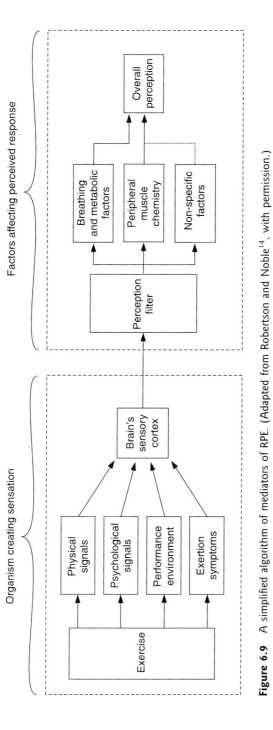

Figure 6.9 A simplified algorithm of mediators of RPE. (Adapted from Robertson and Noble[14], with permission.)

failure is usually due to the need to follow a rigorous scientific method. RPE is no exception to this rule, except for the fact that its rigorous method of use is relatively simple to apply 'in the field'. As it is such a simple-looking scale, often pasted onto a piece of cardboard, it can be used incorrectly, thus invalidating the results. Just because it is simple in use and in appearance does not mean that one can overlook the importance of following a structured procedure for its use. It does not require lengthy impractical calibrations and can stand alone as a response measurement unaffected by many environmental or psychological elements which often need to be controlled or calibrated.[13]

A good example is that sometimes it is difficult in the field to control for such factors as temperature and emotional state on the heart.[13] This example is especially true in the area of health-based exercise, in which non-athletic and newcomer clients are unfamiliar with being clinically measured. However, because the RPE scale is a very 'soft' tool it provides little offence or worry about the outcome. The simple fact of measuring heart rate or blood pressure, as most doctors will confirm, can create an emotional arousal in itself (see the case report below), often termed the 'white coat effect'. Other factors which can affect normal responses to heart rate and even oxygen uptake during exercise are medications, such as beta blockers used by people with high blood pressure or CHD patients. A classic study by Davies and Sargeant[15] (Figure 6.10) showed that RPE was unaffected by heart rate controlling medications, which has important implications for exercise testing and prescription, especially in patient populations (see Chapters 7 and 11).

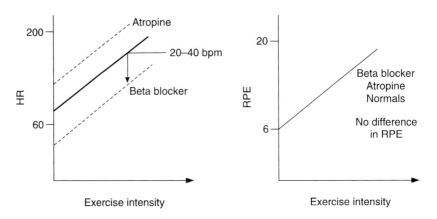

Figure 6.10 The independence of RPE to the effects of cardiovascular controlling mechanisms. (Adapted from Davies and Sergeant[15] and Ekblom et al.[16])

Case report

An active and experienced female exerciser attended for a consultation and assessment. In acknowledging that she had once been a nurse, it was very surprising that she became incredibly anxious when asked to wear a chest strap connected to a simple three-lead ECG monitor for a cycle test. Not only was she a nurse, but had been a specialist working on a coronary care unit. Unfortunately the sight of an ECG trace brought back horrendous memories of trauma in patients she had cared for more than 10 years ago. Such anxiety raised her heart rate above 110 bpm before she even started pedalling, but the RPE scale aided as a back-up to give a good idea of her exercise response. In this case the use of a more simple heart rate monitor should have been used, and highlighted the importance of describing to the client, prior to testing, not just what was going to be measured but how it would be measured and ensuring that substitute measurement tools were available – in this case the more simple heart rate monitor and the RPE scale.

Main points for correct usage of RPE

There are six key factors in ensuring that RPE is used correctly in order to produce valid results:

1. A standardized set of instructions in following points 2–5 below.
2. It should clearly be seen and in full view of the client at all times.
3. Explanation of the scale, why it is used and what it measures.
4. Acknowledging an integrated response (e.g. combined legs, arms, breathing, etc.) or specific body segment response (e.g. used during weight training).
5. Anchoring the sensations of the lowest and highest ratings.
6. Habituation (familiarization/experience).

1. Standardized instruction

In order to ensure that a client uses the scale in the same way each time, so that results are reproducible (reliable), it is important that the same set of instructions are always given. This is especially true, both in an assessment or programme monitoring situation, if two different exercise professionals are using it with the same group of clients or patients.

2. Clearly in full view at all times

It is important that the client or patient can read the chart easily (do they need to wear their glasses?). Before using it, simply ask the client to read the chart from where they will be exercising, much in the same way as they would be asked during an eye test.

3. Explain the scale

Make it clear that this scale is a measure of how hard they are finding the activity *now*. It is an opportunity for them to give a rating to you the assessor and, at any time they feel a change in how they are finding the activity, they should inform you (the assessor) of their new rating. Explain that the scale's lowest level is level 6 and the highest or hardest rating is level 20 (see point 5, anchoring).

4. Integrated or specific location rating

In most cases, typically aerobic activities, the client is asked to give an integrated (all-over feeling) response. Such a response is how all their muscles feel, any levels of pain or ache, breathing, and any other sensations they can feel all put together to give one rating or response. In some instances where it is necessary to find out how a particular muscle group feels (e.g. during weight training or muscle/joint rehabilitation exercises), it may be necessary to gain an RPE for that particular body area.

5. Anchoring the top and bottom of the scale

This process, probably the most important of all the instructions, enables the client to create an association with the lowest and highest exertion levels.

To anchor the lowest rating (rating 6 – no exertion at all), the client should be told that level 6 is a rating they would give if they were sitting back quietly and comfortably in a chair ('sitting in a comfortable chair sipping on their favourite drink').

To anchor the highest ratings (18–20 – maximal exertion), the client should be asked to think back to the hardest they could have imagined exerting themselves, possibly struggling to catch their breath and their whole body feeling completely exhausted and weakened by some physical effort. Some females may associate this with childbirth. Explain to them that if this chart was in front of them at that time, then this is the rating they would have given. Anchoring this end of the scale is slightly more difficult than anchoring the lower end because people's personal perception of maximal effort can vary, but the one benefit is that the scale is thus individualized, with limits set by the client's own perceptions.

6. Habituation

As with any tool, the more people become familiar with it, the better and more effective it becomes. It has even been recommended with patients after a heart attack or heart surgery in the early stages of their hospital (in-patient) stay. From the point when patients become mobile on the hospital ward to participation in a subsequent activity programme with a rehabilitation exercise group, they will become familiar with the scale and use it as a guide.

Different methods of applying RPE

RPE can be applied with three different methods:

1. The *estimation* method.
2. The *production* method.
3. Working to a *preferred* RPE.

1. The estimation method

The estimation method is the most traditional and most widely used application of RPE,[6] in which the exercising client or patient gives an RPE in response to a given intensity of exercise. This is known as a 'passive' use of RPE, where the person is focusing on performing a specific task or predetermined workrate (e.g. cycle watts, walking or running speed) and they then give a rating of their feeling of exertion in response to performing this task.

2. The production method

The production method is a more contemporary application of RPE, in which the client works to a predetermined RPE or is prescribed to work at a set RPE. This is known as an 'active' use of RPE, where RPE becomes the focus of establishing one's effort, as opposed to a passive RPE response to a given task or workrate as described above.[17,18] The prescribed RPE is often based on the estimated RPE response to a given workrate from a treadmill or exercise cycle test.

It has been shown in some studies that when an individual is asked to work to a specific RPE in order to replicate an effort from a previous testing situation, they will tend to produce slightly less effort.[19] If these findings become more conclusive, then this lower effort production will possibly allow for a margin of safety when prescribing exercise to patients with heart disease, especially when the prescribed effort production is based on the RPE response from a graded exercise stress test.

3. The preferred exertion method

The preferred exertion method is the most contemporary application for using RPE and it involves allowing the individual to work to a level at which they feel more comfortable. Recent research in this area has used the 15-point (6–20) RPE scale alongside a 'feeling' scale which measures a score from −5 (displeasure) to +5 (pleasure).[20] It applies a similar process to the production method above, where the individual actively works to a specified RPE. The more highly trained experienced exerciser or athlete may be content to work to higher intensities (RPE 13, 14, 15 or even 16), at which they are also more physiologically equipped to tolerate and sustain such levels. The less experienced or newcomer to the exercise arena may be more comfortable at lower intensities (RPE 10–12).

It was shown by Eston et al.[20] that even at the lower preferred intensities, individuals still worked to levels which would improve cardiorespiratory fitness in line with accepted guidelines (see Chapters 1, 7 and 8). The lower intensity concept also dovetails well with recommendations for newcomers to exercise, as outlined in Chapter 3, where the focus is on adopting the behaviour of regular participation first and then at a later point focusing more concern on specific physiologically beneficial levels of intensity.

Blood pressure

Blood pressure is an essential mechanism in the body, for without it there is no circulation and thus no delivery of life-giving oxygen and nutrients to the vital organs. Blood pressure is typically measured by a device called a sphygmomanometer and the units of measure are in millimetres of mercury (mmHg).

Measurement considers two elements of blood pressure – the systolic pressure and the diastolic pressure. Systole is the period where the heart muscle contracts and ejects the blood into the arteries and the pressure rises at this point. Once this contraction of the heart is complete there is a brief rest period in between heart beats, when the heart is refilling the ventricles, known as diastole, where the blood flow briefly loses momentum and thus there is a brief drop in pressure. When blood pressure is measured, the systolic pressure is the peak pressure during the contraction of the heart and the diastolic pressure is the lower pressure occurring in between beats of the heart.

A typical healthy resting systolic pressure ranges from 100 to 140 mmHg and a healthy diastolic pressure from 60 to 90 mmHg. If either the systolic or the diastolic rise above these levels, at rest, then an individual may be classed as having high blood pressure or hypertension.

Exercising blood pressure

During the activities or exercise intensities recommended in this book, systolic blood pressure should rise in proportion to the amount of effort, in a similar manner to exercising heart rate. This pressure rise, depending on the intensity and the resting systolic pressure, can typically reach 200 mmHg. At the same time, however, diastolic pressure should remain unchanged, not rising more than 10 mmHg or possibly even dropping slightly.[4] Only within the first 30–60 seconds of initiating exercise should there ever be a drop in systolic pressure.[21] After this point, with increasing levels of exercise intensity there should be a corresponding rise in systolic pressure (Figure 6.11). A failure of systolic pressure to rise or even worse a drop with an increase in exercise intensity is often used as an indication of the heart failing to pump effectively. During exercise stress tests of cardiac patients, this criterion is used as one of the main reasons to stop the test immediately.[5]

The rise in systolic pressure during exercise is due to both the strength and rate of contraction of the heart muscle, and as long as the diastolic does not rise too much it means that the blood vessels have dilated and the heart is pumping effectively. During rest, a rise in either systolic or diastolic pressure is due to the fact that the blood vessels have constricted (known as vasoconstriction) causing extra pressure against which the heart has to pump. Vasoconstriction at rest can result from an emotional response (stress) and/or related hormonal changes or from a change in blood biochemistry due to dietary or other acquired illness factors.

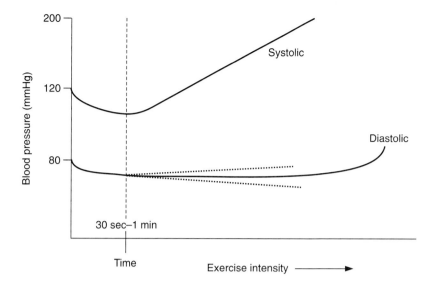

Figure 6.11 Typical blood pressure response to increasing intensities of exercise. Note that in the early onset of exercise (30 sec to 1 min) there may be a drop in blood pressure from the combined adjustment of decreasing blood flow to the gut area and its increase to the exercising combined muscles. (Adapted from Raven et al.[21])

Exercising blood pressure is most easily measured during cycle ergometry because the arm can be kept virtually still. Before the exercise professional attempts to measure blood pressure during exercise it is paramount that they are highly skilled at measuring blood pressure at rest. There are very few automatic or electronic sphygmomanometers that work accurately during exercise and thus a manual mercury sphygmomanometer is recommended.

References

1. Borg, G. (1982) Pscychophysical bases of perceived exertion. *Med Sci. Sports Exerc.*, **14**, 377–381.
2. Astrand, P.O. and Rodahl, K. (1986) *Text Book of Work Physiology: Physiological Bases of Exercise*, McGraw-Hill, New York.
3. Robinson, S. (1938) Experimental studies of physical fitness in relation to age. *Arbeitphysiol.*, **10**, 251.
4. Astrand, I., Astrand, P.-O. and Rodahl, K. (1959) Maximal heart rate during work in older men. *J. Appl. Physiol.*, **14**, 562.
5. Londeree, B.R. and Moeschberger, M.L. (1984) Influence of age and other factors on maximal heart rate. *J. Cardiac. Rehab.*, **41**, 44–49.
6. Noble, B. and Robertson, R. (1996) *Perceived Exertion, Human Kinetics*, Champaign, IL.
7. American College of Sports Medicine (1995) *Guidelines for Exercise Testing and Prescription*, 5th edn, Williams and Wilkins, Philadelphia.

8. Coats, A. McGee, H., Stokes, H. and Thompson, D. (1995) *Guidelines for Cardiac Rehabilitation*, The British Association for Cardiac Rehabilitation, Blackwell, Oxford.

9. Pollock, M. and Schmidt, D. (1995) *Heart Disease and Rehabilitation*, Human Kinetics, Champaign, Il.

10. American Association for Cardiovascular and Pulmonary Rehabilitation (1995) *Guidelines for Cardiac Rehabilitation Programmes*, Human Kinetics, Champaign, IL.

11. Eston, R. and Connolly, D. (1996) The use of ratings of perceived exertion for exercise prescription in patients receiving beta-blocker therapy. *Sports Med.*, **21**(3), 176–190.

12. Borg, G.E. (1985) *An Introduction to Borg's RPE Scale*, Ithaca, New York.

13. Dishman, R.K. (1994) Prescribing exercise intensity for healthy adults using perceived exertion. *Med. Sci. Sports Exerc.*, **26**, 1087–1094.

14. Robertson, R.J. and Noble, B.J. (1997) Perception of physical exertion: methods, mediators and applications. *Exerc. Sports Sci. Rev.*, **25**, 407–452.

15. Davies, C.T. and Sargeant A.J. (1979). The effects of atropine and practolol on the perception of exertion during treadmill exercise. *Ergonomics*, **22**, 1141–1146.

16. Ekblom, B., Goldbarg, A.N., Kilbom, A. and Astrand P.-O. (1972) Effects of atropine and propanolol on the oxygen transport system during exercise in man. *Scand. J. Clin. Lab. Invest.*, **33**, 175.

17. Dunbar, C.C., Robertson, R.J., Baun, R. *et al.* (1992) The validity of regulating exercise intensity by ratings of perceived exertion. *Med. Sci. Sports Exerc.*, **24**, 94–99.

18. Eston, R.G., Davies, B.L. and Williams, J.G. (1987) Use of ratings of perceived effort to control exercise intensity in young healthy adults. *Eur. J. Appl. Physiol.*, **56**, 222–224.

19. Byrne, C. and Eston, R.G. (1997) Use of ratings of perceived exertion to regulate exercise intensity: a study using effort estimation and effort production. Conference Proceedings of The British Association of Sport and Exercise Sciences, York, September.

20. Eston, R., Parfitt, G. and Tucker, R.J. (1997) Ratings of perceived exertion and psychological effect during preferred exercise intensity in high- and low-active men. Conference Proceedings of The British Association of Sport and Exercise Sciences, York, September.

21. Raven, P.B., Potts, J.T. and Xiangrong, S. (1997) Baroreflex regulation of blood pressure during dynamic exercise. *Exerc. Sports Sci. Rev.*, **25**, 365–389.

7

Prescribing activity and exercise for health and fitness

What are people's activity choices?

Setting the intensity of activity – the key element

Increasing activity in daily living versus the traditional 'three times per week for 20 minutes' message

Performing daily activity tasks using ratings of perceived exertion and heart rate

Ensuring a clear understanding of the concept of exercise workrate

Establishing exercise workrates or target heart rates from ratings of perceived exertion during a submaximal exercise cycle test

Chapter summary

References

The first six chapters have offered the reader some of the underlying health and physiological principles of cardiovascular activity along with the applied experiences of the authors. These chapters have formed the 'tool bag' of this book and this chapter and those to follow are thus about using 'the tools' effectively for the benefit of the client.

The first part of this chapter will simply extend much of the concepts of daily living activity outlined in Chapters 1, 2 and 3 and look at how to assist people from a simple advisory approach. The second part is more closely related to Chapters 8, 9 and 12 on designing more structured exercise regimens using heart rate and ratings of perceived exertion. Chapters 8 and 9 will take the structured exercise assessment and programming concept even further with the use of specific exercise ergometers (machines). Chapter 12 is devoted to how to effectively *deliver* a full consultation, which provides the framework for linking and 'packaging up' the information from all the other 11 chapters of this book.

What are people's activity choices?

One of the most important matters to respect in any person is that they have freedom of choice. Professor Stephen Blair (a leading authority of the U.S. Centres for Disease Control and the American College of Sports Medicine) put it very simply at his 1997 'Keynote' lecture to the British Association of Sports and Exercise Sciences... people have three choices when it comes to being more active and taking up health-related exercise:

1. They have the choice to do nothing,
2. They can pursue the traditional approach of exercising at least three times per week, continuously for 20–60 minutes with large muscle groups at an intensity of 60–85% of maximum heart rate, or 50–80% of $\dot{V}O_{2max}$ or at an RPE of 12–14 (as noted in Chapters 1, 4–6, 8 and 9), and/or
3. They can create activity interventions into their daily lifestyle (see Chapter 1 on the U.S. Surgeon General's report and Chapter 2, reference to Pate et al.[33]) which should equate to lower levels of movement intensity possibly sustained for at least 10 minutes but accumulating up to 30 minutes per day.

Setting the intensity of activity – the key element

In the descriptions above of prescribed activity, whether through the traditional message or the more contemporary daily activity message, the question least resolved is 'How hard should I actually be working?' The answer is that *this is different for everyone*. A misconception is that many individuals think that activity and exercise have to be hard or uncomfortable to be effective. Of course, if you are training for the Olympic 1500 metres race, then you would have to train to learn to cope with the pain of the final lap. If, however, activity and exercise/training are for health, there is no need to push to this degree; in fact, it would be considered unhealthy and risky to do so.

The daily activity message focuses on the idea that if one is active at lower intensities, the activity must be performed for longer to obtain similar health benefits (but not necessarily fitness) than if one were to go harder for shorter periods. Chapter 1 (Figure 1.3) highlighted that health but not necessarily fitness gains could be obtained at activity intensities lower than 50–55% of one's aerobic capacity ($\dot{V}O_{2max}$). What level is 50–55% $\dot{V}O_{2max}$ and how much can it vary from one person to the next? As shown in Chapters 4 and 5, if an elite marathon runner exerts himself to 60% of his capacity, which for him is fairly steady and easy, it is equivalent to a running pace of 6 minutes per mile. For most people to be able to run one mile in six minutes would be far beyond their maximal capacity. At the other end of the scale, if an obese cardiac patient exerts themselves to 60% of their capacity, it is quite likely to be equivalent to what most people consider a very slow walking pace of 30 minutes per mile. The important point is that in both these examples, the marathon runner and the cardiac patient are exercising to the same level *relative* to their own ability, even though there is a wide gulf between the *absolute* intensity as measured in minutes per mile. The cardiac patient working to 60% of their capacity is enough (see Chapter 11) to confer health benefits and improve their VO_{2max} – assuming that a regular (*frequency*) programme is followed for *durations* in excess of 15 minutes. The marathon runner will, however, have to train at 75–90% of their capacity to at least maintain their existing performance ability. These concepts are important for clearly understanding Chapter 9. Chapter 5 describes the concept of *training status* as being as important to setting intensity, as is overall aerobic capacity.

Intensity is the key, and a great deal of the remainder of this book will specifically deal with this fact. If the intensity is set appropriately, then all clients can gain a sense of achievement with regard to the other prescription elements of how long (*duration*) and how often (*frequency*). Professor Blair's choices 2 and 3, given above, both contained elements of duration, frequency and intensity – the key ingredients of any activity or exercise prescription. Duration and frequency must also be individualized in order to establish a progression, but the framework for these is generally established by the fact that if an individual is following the minimum of 20 minutes three times per week, it must be at an intensity of at least 55–60% of their aerobic capacity.

The activity model for improving health (i.e. blood pressure, cholesterol), accumulating 30 minutes per day can be done at intensities ranging as low as by 40% and up to the typical exercise levels of 55–75% of aerobic capacity. As one can see, the duration is a function of intensity; get the intensity incorrect and the beneficial duration may not be achievable. Frequency depends on time availability, familiarity and allowing the body to adapt to being able to exercise more vigorously. In the initial stages, to overcome the expected muscle stiffness when just starting a programme, two times per week, with enough days in between to allow the stiffness or minor aches to resolve, may be suitable and then progressing to three times per week. Unless a person is highly trained or an athlete, there should be at least 2–3 rest days per week to allow the body to recover and restore its energy stores.

A key benefit of a properly conducted exercise consultation, as described later in this chapter and in Chapters 8 and 9, is the effective establishment of the activity or exercise intensity. It is possible for people to find the right intensity on their own through *trial and error*, but during this period of trial and error how does one know whether it is safe and/or effective? From the authors' experience most people will start off too hard too soon. The trial and error approach to establishing the correct intensity often results in some degree of failure because the individual is unable to meet the standard duration target. Chapter 3 highlighted people's sense of failure and dropout in the early stages of attending an exercise centre. Is there a possible link between ineffective guidance, or possibly no guidance at all, and the 60% dropout rate? (This is answered later in the chapter, or the sections on adherence in Chapter 3 may be read again.)

One of the best examples of observing our inability to set the correct pace is to ask a group of children to run around a soccer pitch (or a field) three times. The children will race off as fast as they can and before they complete one lap, 80–90% of them will have greatly slowed or had to walk. Only 10–20% of the children who have been genetically endowed with endurance abilities will be able to sustain a steady running pace.

Remember those cross-country runs at school in the pouring rain; for most kids it was an unpleasant experience but for a few they seemed to be able to keep going, with a great sense of achievement. Did these children with endurance ability receive any more coaching than the rest of the class? Probably not!

In reviewing the consultation documents of the 4000 individuals assessed by the authors, those who required exercise for preventative health reasons were mainly those who stated: 'I am not the sporty type and was never good at games or sport at school when I was younger.' It is strongly believed that because they were slightly put off from traditional school physical education they never properly learned the concept of pacing or gaining a beneficial feeling from physical training. The intensity was probably too hard for them to maintain and achieve any feeling of success. Sports/games which required skill, balance and coordination probably also failed them, but being physically active does not require highly skilled movements.

Pacing is something which needs to be learned and an assessment of a client's endurance or aerobic capacity, coupled with a recent history of how much they train, provides a means of establishing the right pace (see also Chapters 8 and 9). It is possible that humans do not possess an innate concept of pace because our purely biological rationale for running is to get ourselves quickly out of danger, which was required when humans used to survive by hunting for food. Now that most people's lives in the Western world require little physical exertion to achieve survival, we are no longer steadily activating our muscles throughout the day. To substitute for this loss of activity and possibly the inherent competition to hunt and survive, humans have invented recreation of shorter bouts of activity in what is now known as leisure time, in order to expend similar levels of energy. Unfortunately, as highlighted in Chapters 1 and 2, as the Western world has become more technically advanced, more people are less active and more sedentary (70–80% of the population) and are not making an effort to replace this reduced energy expenditure with purposeful activity. Because many lack regular daily exertion of their muscles, the concept of pace to the average person is now even more unnatural.

The aim of the daily activity message is an attempt to restore continual lower intensity but constant movement now lacking, which our ancestors from the agricultural era gained from ploughing, planting and harvesting by hand. Many underdeveloped cultures still live in this era and have much lower levels of heart disease than industrialized nations, even though they may smoke and may not have the resources to choose a healthy diet like those in the Western industrialized societies.

Increasing activity in daily living versus the traditional 'three times per week for 20 minutes' message

The essential elements of the *three times per week for at least 20 minutes* message has now been established for more than 30 years, with variations on this theme being added over time. As noted in Chapter 2, this message has, however, only been taken up by about 20–25% of the population of those Western societies most affected by sedentary lifestyles. This 20–25% group are those who are either self-disciplined enough to exercise on their own or who regularly attend exercise classes, a gym, or clubs for sports, running, athletics and outdoor pusuits. By no means does this make the aims of this message redundant, but there is a strong question mark over how possible it is to get the remaining 75–80% of the population to adopt this behaviour of a regular structured exercise regimen. For many people this would require a large transition, possibly an unacceptable change, from their freely chosen lifestyle. Chapter 3 acknowledged many of the actual and perceived barriers to such behavioural change.

In those who are able to adopt the three times per week for 20 minutes message it is important to ensure that both their programming and supervision are to a standard which provides encouragement, progression and adaptability to their ever-changing physical, psychological and social needs. Without this, many people are likely to drop out, as shown by statistics of the UK fitness industry showing attrition rates of up to 60% within 6 months. Chapter 3 stated, however, that the rate of dropout was significantly decreased when quality guidance and supervision were given. The final part of this present chapter and through to Chapter 12 is specifically designed to equip the practitioner with the tools to achieve quality guidance and programme adaptability.

The *lifestyle activity intervention message*, as noted in Professor Blair's third choice, is the more contemporary goal of government programmes in Britain, the USA, Canada, Australia and other similar developed societies. In all these countries, as described in Chapter 2, there is now a conclusive link between heart disease and inactivity, so much so that even low doses of regular activity can confer significant health benefits and changes in CHD risk factors (blood pressure, cholesterol, diabetes, fibrinogen). This message addresses a more adoptable approach by asking: What is the least people can do to gain some benefit? This message is being seriously entertained and promoted by government-backed public health programmes – in the USA by the Centers for Disease Control and Prevention (CDC) and in England by the Health Education Authority (HEA). Both these agencies have linked themselves to accredited research-based institutions; The American College of Sports Medicine and The British Association of Sports and Exercise Sciences.

The lifestyle activity intervention message is a concept which requires a less abrupt behavioural change. The aims are to show people how to be more active during their normal daily routines, with the simple fact that the more a person engages their muscles, joints and circulation, as opposed to sitting or standing, then the body's metabolic rate is at least raised to a state to confer some beneficial adaptations.

Ideas and initiatives of advice for increasing daily activity

The following examples are just a few which may give health professionals and exercise advisers some ideas to discuss with their clients or patients. The main aim is to discuss with the client where in their daily living are they actually using their arms and legs and then to make adjustments so they simply create opportunities to do more of these movements. The client therefore sees less of a disciplined approach, with fewer potential perceived behavioural change barriers that otherwise might impact on their normal daily routines.

The car at the supermarket concept

How much time do you spend driving around trying to find a parking spot as close to the supermarket as possible? Often 5 minutes, maybe even 7 to 10 minutes, waiting for someone else to vacate their spot? If you park at the far end of the car park and spend the 5–7 minutes walking to the supermarket, you would arrive at the door in the same amount of time but will have expended up to 50 more calories. There is then the 5-minute walk back to the car, which is probably a little more than the 50 calories because you have had to push the shopping trolley. In total you have only lost 5 minutes of your day but expended twice the calories than if you had used a parking spot nearer to the supermarket.

The shopping mall escalator or elevator/lift

All shops have stairs and yet people are quite happy to queue to get onto an escalator, even when it is going down. Again, the journey by using the stairs would have not taken much longer than the slow-moving escalator and you will have expended energy.

The 10-minute walk three times per day

Is it really too much to get up in the morning 10 minutes earlier and simply go for a walk prior to going to work; and instead of the coffee break at 10.45 am to take a walk and then again at lunch? You do not have to break into a sweat. Simply having your muscles, joints and circulation being moved for 10 minutes without stopping is something 80% of the population are not doing. Over the course of a day, this adds up to 30 minutes (150–300 extra calories burned). Over a week this is 1000–2000 extra calories burned.

Gardening with manual rather than power tools

In Britain, gardens on average are smaller than those in America and yet many people use the same power tools. Is it not better to burn a few extra calories each weekend over the rest of your life and activate your muscles, joints and circulation, rather than finishing a little more quickly so that you may have longer in the chair to watch television, where you sit with your muscles and joints idle? The US Surgeon General's report rates idleness on a par with health risks of smoking. In fact, idleness and being sedentary may possibly have a greater impact on the US population than the effects of smoking. As the US Centres for Disease Control reports, only about 30% of the population smoke but over 70% of the population are sedentary. Furthermore, a sedentary lifestyle couched in front of a television could be as damaging socially as it is physically.

The use of public transport

With the environmentalists confronting us for using our cars too much, this policy can have a double impact on public health. Whenever convenience and time are less of a priority, the simple walk from the house or park and ride station, to the bus or train, and the walk at the other end to your destination, is similar to the car at the supermarket example given above.

The suggestions above are very simple tasks which more engage people's muscles, joints and circulation and, although not to a level which may improve fitness, the accumulated expended calories over weeks, months and years can have a profound effect on one's health. It will be interesting to see if the new public health message is adopted in a larger proportion of the 75–80% of the population who are at present highly sedentary. Whether or not this can be achieved may be questioned, but those who do take it up will benefit.

Does the new lifestyle activity intervention and public health message need to confront people more in order to be effective?

It may be a fact that an even tougher approach needs to be taken, similar to that of the anti-smoking message, to stimulate more active movement into people's lives. With smoking it is known that raising the cost of cigarettes or printing health warning messages on cigarette packages have probably not affected behaviour change. The warning labels are there more for legal protection of the tobacco companies, a fact which has been highlighted by the very public legal cases against them. The question being asked is: Did the tobacco companies know smoking was a health hazard before they were required to put health warning messages on adverts and packaging? What has impacted on smokers is the growing social inacceptability of smoking which confronts smokers daily. Non-smoking policies in buildings, on trains and buses, on airlines, in restaurants, in people's own homes, etc., have created a growing barrier for smokers. Just think what might happen if a majority of pubs in Britain had no-smoking policies.

Imagine if there were similar policies which restricted the use of cars, escalators, elevators/lifts, hours of television watched or computer games played, hours at work sitting rather than standing and moving, and no car parking for parents within half a mile of a school. It may infringe on people's rights to invoke such drastic policies, but if health advisers (doctors, nurses and all health promoters) could stimulate people to invoke such policies on themselves, the effects on public health would be significant. This was noted in Chapter 2, where it mentioned Professor Claude Bouchard's work showing the average person in the 1990s expends 500 fewer calories in their daily life compared with the average person in the 1950s. Five hundred calories for the average person is equivalent to a continuous very brisk walk or steady jog for 30–40 minutes.

The key culprits of the mounting lack of calories expended in a day are all the various labour-saving devices or increasing amounts of sedentary pastimes (cars, home and garden appliances, automated manufacturing devices, escalators and lifts, the need for children's safe transport to school, television, computers and computer games). People may not realize, until they are shown, that just a little use of these labour-saving devices over the 16 hours they are awake can easily amount to expending 500 fewer calories per day as compared to a person in the 1950s.

A case in point

An advance in working conditions which may decrease activity and increase the risk factors of heart disease in Britain could be as follows:

An interesting scenario in Britain involving rubbish collection services is the provision to many households of what is known as a 'wheelie bin', a large rubbish bin (garbage can) on wheels. Not only does it ease the work (reduces energy expended) involved in carrying the bags to the end of people's drives, but the bins are specially designed so that the refuse operators do not have to exert themselves to pick them up. There is a special lift on the back of the collection truck which picks up the bins and empties them, thus removing any physical muscular effort from the operators. Some health and safety inspectors may state that they are preventing back problems in the workers, but opposingly these workers will have greatly reduced energy expenditure and lower levels of daily circulation. The lack of muscular work will in fact reduce their fitness, so that potentially when they are performing other physical tasks (e.g. gardening), they may be more prone to back and joint problems due to the reduction of daily activity in their work. The amount of energy expended in lifting the rubbish bags from the ground and throwing them into the truck, over four or five hours, is a good level of daily energy expenditure, enough to confer a preventative effect noted in Chapter 2 regarding the causes of heart disease. The reduced energy expenditure from the easing of the work by the use of wheelie bins will probably not be counterbalanced by a reduction in the workers' daily energy intake of food. In order for these men and women to make up for the calories lost, they would probably have to exercise vigorously every day for over an hour without stopping.

Getting sedentary people to be more active in their daily lives may eventually lead to their desire to take up more formal or structured activities of exercise once the initial health benefits are noticed. Although such individuals will have fulfilled the minimum requirements, the engaging of more vigorous activity can bring added benefits. Changes in cholesterol and blood pressure are the most widely acknowledged of those monitored by the family doctor, and have been shown in Chapter 2 to be strong outcome measures following an increase in daily energy expenditure, with further benefits from more vigorous structured activity.

Advising clients on increased daily activity

It would seem sensible for venues of health-related activity, including doctors' practices, leisure centres, health promotion units and even hospitals, to consider offering advisory services on activity in daily living. It is quite feasible for this to be done in group sessions, to which the clients have been recommended by their family doctor or nurse.

Accumulating enough activity to effect health

The simple aim of the advice is to identify, as suggested earlier, any possible ways people can carry out daily tasks, or going to and from typical daily tasks, using their arms and legs as much of the time as possible. The aim is to get people to accumulate activity points where for each minute they are 'active' they get 5 points (approximately 5 extra calories burned). In order to achieve noticeable benefit they should aim to accumulate 1500–2000 activity points per week. Obviously, double points should be given if they accumulate extra points as a result of participating in more structured exercise. In many cases it may be found that those who are more active in their daily living could easily accumulate more points than those who think they are doing well by performing two vigorous exercise sessions per week and then feel justified to take it easy.

If individuals participate in less than 120 minutes of regular more vigorous structured exercise per week, it may be still important for them to consider being active during the rest of their daily life. This is not to say that less than 120 minutes is not beneficial, because the dose response concept states that *anything is better than nothing* and 120 minutes is a reasonable amount. Although, participating in less frequent exercise and fitness regimens can still be beneficial because they can have a 'knock-on' effect on the quality of the rest of one's life (physically, socially, psychologically), as highlighted in Chapters 1–3. The health benefits of exercise programmes may not always be directly attributable to increased fitness, but that increased fitness has allowed an individual to perform their normal daily and leisure routines with more vigour, at more pace, with confidence and control, and thus conferring both a physical and psychological health benefit. Furthermore, those who are concious about one aspect of their health (i.e their fitness) may also become more conscious about other health aspects (food, alcohol, rest and stress), again an example where exercise and fitness are catalysts to other health behaviours and not necessarily the direct mechanism of improved health.

Performing daily activity tasks using ratings of perceived exertion and heart rate

Ensure an understanding of Chapter 6 before proceeding.

Some individuals may wish to monitor more closely the intensity to which they perform their daily activities (e.g. walking the dog, walking to pick the children up from school, walking to town or to the newspaper shop, gardening). It must first be determined to what level the individual wishes to work and whether they are interested in achieving:

(a) simply some moderate health gains (affecting blood pressure and cholesterol),
(b) health and fitness gains, which may have a more profound effect on their physical shape as well as the health gains noted in point (a),
(c) maintainenance of the *status quo*, at least, and preventing any further decline in health and reducing some of the effects of ageing.

Structuring intensity for moderate health gain

In the case of point (a), the person's whole body or integrated rating of perceived exertion (RPE) during any given task should be 9–11, which equates to around 40–50% of their aerobic capacity. It is recommended to give clients pocket-sized RPE scales. The RPE scale (see Figure 6.8) can be reduced by a photocopier and then plastic laminated. Heart rate can also be used where the client performs their activity task to a level of approximately 50–60% of their maximal heart rate (50–60% of $220-\text{age}$) or maximal heart rate (HR_{max}) reserve (Table 7.1, or see Chapter 6 for clarification). There is obviously some difficulty in measuring heart rate, unless the client is willing to purchase a wireless chest strap heart rate monitor (cost approximately £50 UK or $80 USA), widely available at most sports and cycle shops. It is important to consider the other constraints of using age-predicted HR_{max}, as noted in Chapter 6. A final measurement may be what is known as a *talking threshold*. If a person is unable to talk comfortably while performing their task, then their ventilation rate is beyond that considered to be mild to moderate exertion.

The heart rate reserve method is based on the difference between a persons's resting heart rate and their HR_{max}. The latter can either be estimated by age ($220-\text{age}$) or from a maximal test. Please note the caution given earlier regarding the safety of performing maximal tests. Table 7.1 performs the following calculation:

$$\text{HR reserve} = 60\% \text{ and } 80\% \text{ of } (HR_{max} - HR_{rest}) + HR_{rest}$$

Table 7.1 Calculating 60–80% of HR_{max} reserve*. (Adapted from Karvonen et al.[1])

Resting HR:	Age 20 or HR_{max} 200		Age 25 or HR_{max} 195		Age 30 or HR_{max} 190		Age 35 or HR_{max} 185		Age 40 or HR_{max} 180		Age 45 or HR_{max} 175	
	60%	80%	60%	80%	60%	80%	60%	80%	60%	80%	60%	80%
40	136	168	133	164	130	160	127	156	124	152	121	148
45	138	169	135	165	132	161	129	157	126	153	123	149
50	140	170	137	166	134	162	131	158	128	154	125	150
55	142	171	139	167	136	163	133	159	130	155	127	151
60	144	172	141	168	138	164	135	160	132	156	129	152
65	146	173	143	169	140	165	137	161	134	157	131	153
70	148	174	145	170	142	166	139	162	136	158	133	154
75	150	175	147	171	144	167	141	163	138	159	135	155
80	152	176	149	172	146	168	143	164	140	160	137	156
85	154	177	151	173	148	169	145	165	142	161	139	157
90	156	178	153	174	150	170	147	166	144	162	141	158
95	158	179	155	175	152	171	149	167	146	163	143	159
100	160	180	157	176	154	172	151	168	148	164	145	160
105	162	181	159	177	156	173	153	169	150	165	147	161

Resting HR:	Age 50 or HR_{max} 170		Age 55 or HR_{max} 165		Age 60 or HR_{max} 160		Age 65 or HR_{max} 155		Age 70 or HR_{max} 150		Age 75 or HR_{max} 145	
	60%	80%	60%	80%	60%	80%	60%	80%	60%	80%	60%	80%
40	118	144	115	140	112	136	109	132	107	128	104	124
45	120	145	117	141	114	137	111	133	109	129	106	125
50	122	146	119	142	116	138	113	134	111	130	108	
55	124	147	121	143	118	139	115	135	113		110	
60	126	148	123	144	120	140	117		115		112	
65	128	149	125	145	122	141	119		117		114	
70	130	150	127	146	124	142	121		119			
75	132	151	129	147	126	143	123					
80	134	152	131	148	128	144						
85	136	153	133	149	130	145						
90	138	154	135	150	132							
95	140	155	137	151	134							
100	142	156	139	152	136							
105	144	157	141	153	138							

*Instructions:

Determine a person's resting heart rate and find it down the left-hand column.

Read across to either their age or the maximal heart rate determined during a test.

The value under the 60% column is 60% of their maximal heart rate reserve and ditto for the 80% column.

For non-beta-blocked cardiac rehabilitation patients, the HR_{max} achieved or their HR at the onset of ischaemia in their stress test can be used as their maximum heart rate irrespective of age.

Working between 60% and 80% of HR_{max} reserve is the level recommended by the American College of Sports Medicine.

A start to structuring exercise intensity for health, fitness and physical appearance

With regard to point (b) above, it is important to remember that the client is aiming to exert themselves to higher levels. In this case possible closer attention, professional guidance and more specific understanding of heart rate and RPE are required. It may be necessary for the client to perform their own mini-assessment, where they set a specific walking or jogging distance to cover (i.e. 1 or 2 miles). The aim is for them to walk/jog the 1- or 2-mile circuit with a pace eliciting an RPE of 11 or 12 and 13 as an upper limit (approximately 55–65% $\dot{V}O_{2max}$). It is important to acknowledge whether they are using the RPE by the *effort estimation* or the *effort production* method, as outlined in Chapter 6. With effort production the client may tend to work a little less hard in relation to their estimated effort RPE taken from the initial assessment. At this intensity they time how long it takes to cover the distance and practise learning that pace. If every two or three weeks they reassess themselves performing the exact same distance circuit at the same RPE, their time should become a little quicker. If they use a heart rate monitor, then again they can use their heart rate as a standard measurement similar to that of RPE. A target heart rate can be established as above in point (a). At a given heart rate, after a number of weeks, their time to complete the circuit should be quicker. In the period of weeks between assessments, the person should be encouraged to perform a variety of activities or have different walking circuits other than the one used for the assessment, to add variety and interest. It is important to note that if the person has any cardiovascular problems (blood pressure, heart rate affected by medication, an irregular heart rate), then the heart rate guidelines to this point in the chapter will not be valid. Later sections in this chapter and in Chapter 11 describe how atypical heart rates can be adapted. To this extent this shows the strength and independence of RPE as a monitoring tool, as discussed in Chapter 6.

The important concept for people to remember is that it does not really matter what the assessment task is, *as long as it is standardized* either by length, time, RPE or heart rate. For example, a person may be able to measure their improvement by the two flights of stairs at work where, after a period of being more active, they simply feel 'less out of puff' walking from the car park up the stairs to their office. Others may be able to walk up to the top of a certain hill more quickly and get less out of puff. These are examples of assessment tasks which are far more meaningful to the client than their $\dot{V}O_{2max}$ score predicted in the consultation.

In Chapter 12, on the consultation, the importance of recording the client's own means of assessing their improvement is acknowledged. Chapters 8 and 9, however, specifically concentrate on using a predicted $\dot{V}O_{2max}$ score, but where the emphasis is on how this score is used as a tool for establishing beneficial exercise intensities as opposed to telling a client how poor, average or good their fitness is. Further rationale for such an approach is more fully discussed in Chapter 12 with regard to a number of health and fitness measures.

The more structured cardiovascular exercise assessment

With regards to a *health-based* exercise assessment performed by an exercise professional, the authors' preferred mode of assessment is the stationary exercise cycle ergometer. Many of the reasons below are made in comparison to assessing clients with either a motorized treadmill, a timed circuit, shuttle, step test or outdoor activity based assessment. The merits of using the cycle ergometer in *health-based submaximal* assessments are that it:

- allows for the resistance to be initially set to relatively low levels, even lower than their normal walking pace, so that clients with varying fitness levels can all complete a standard time – typically at least 5 minutes,
- may give a great sense of achievement to many who have not exercised for a great number of years or who are recovering from an illness, if they are able to exercise non-stop for 6 minutes, leading to immediate feelings of mastery and self-efficacy, as described in Chapter 3,
- requires a low level of skill, coordination or balance, which almost eliminates any 'learning effect' on assessment results,
- allows for the easy taking of response measurements including heart rate, RPE and blood pressure, without the worry of interference from vigorous body movements,
- allows the client to concentrate more easily on observing their exercise intensity and giving verbal responses without having to concentrate very much on the skill of the activity,
- allows simple adjustment of intensity at any time, by either the assessor or the client,
- ensures that exercise responses are largely independent of body weight, because the body is supported,
- allows the client immediately to choose if they feel the need to slow or stop, as it is simply a matter of stopping pedalling, without the worry of any buttons to push and losing their balance,
- allows the assessor to stay close at all times to remark or observe any expressions or gestures of discomfort or changes in skin pallor.

In Tables 7.2 (METs equivalent cycle chart), 7.3 (METs to daily chores conversion), 7.4 (the Buckley/Lifestyle chart), and 7.5 (METs conversion to walking pace), cycle ergometer workrates (intensities) can be converted into other modes of activity. In these tables, METs are the multiples of resting rate – the oxygen uptake equivalent of 1 MET is 3.5 $ml^{-1}. kg^{-1}. min^{-1}$.

Table 7.2 Energy expenditure during cycle ergometry. (By courtesy of Action Heart, Dudley)

Work rate		Oxygen uptake	METS		
(watts)	(kg. min^{-1})	(litres. min^{-1})	60 kg	75 kg	100 kg
50	300	0.9	4.3	3.4	2.6
100	600	1.5	7.1	5.7	4.3
150	900	2.1	10.0	8.0	6.0
200	1200	2.8	13.3	10.7	8.0
250	1500	3.5	16.7	13.3	10.0
300	1800	4.2	20.0	16.0	12.0

Table 7.3 Energy requirements, in METS, of activities of daily living. (From Ainsworth et al.,[2] 1993, with permission)

Activity	MET value*
Personal care	
Bathing	2.0
Dressing/undressing	2.5
Showering	4.0
Cleaning	
Light, e.g. dusting, vacuuming, changing beds	2.5
Heavy, major, e.g. washing windows, mopping	4.5
Moving furniture	6.0
Sweeping garage	4.0
Light domestic activities	
Washing up, serving food, putting away groceries	2.5
Ironing	2.3
DIY activities	
Carpentry	3.01 – 6.0
Laying carpets/linoleum	4.5
Decorating	4.5
Wiring/plumbing	3.0
Food shopping	
Using trolley	3.5
Walking, standing shopping	2.0 – 2.3
Gardening	
Digging	5.0
Mowing lawn (powered hand-mower)	4.5
Raking	4.0
Shovelling snow	6.0

*See text for definition of METS.

Table 7.4 Exercise intensity equivalents for ergometer cycling, rowing and walking/running (weight corrected)

Cycle work* (watts)	Row rate (500 m pace)	Weight (st.): 7.5–8.5 Weight (kg): 50–55 T'mill (kph)	8.5–9.5 55–60 T'mill (kph)	9.5–10 60–65 T'mill (kph)	10–11 65–70 T'mill (kph)	11–11.5 70–75 T'mill (kph)	11.5–12.5 75–80 T'mill (kph)	12.5–13 80–85 T'mill (kph)	13–14 85–90 T'mill (kph)	14–15 90–95 T'mill (kph)	15–15.5 95–100 T'mill (kph)	15.5–16.5 100–105 T'mill (kph)	16.5–17 105–110 T'mill (kph)
50	3:40	4.39	4.01	3.69	3.41	3.18	2.97	2.79	2.63	2.49	2.36	2.25	2.14
65	3:25	5.71	5.21	4.79	4.44	4.13	3.87	3.63	3.42	3.24	3.07	2.92	2.79
80	3:05	7.02	6.41	5.89	5.46	5.08	4.75	4.47	4.21	3.98	3.78	3.59	3.43
100	2:55	8.78	8.02	7.38	6.83	6.36	5.95	5.59	5.27	4.98	4.73	4.5	4.29
110	2:45	9.65	8.81	8.11	7.51	6.99	6.54	6.14	5.79	5.48	5.2	4.94	4.71
130	2:30	11.41	10.42	9.58	8.87	8.26	7.73	7.26	6.85	6.48	6.14	5.84	5.57
150	2:25	13.17	12.02	11.06	10.24	9.54	8.92	8.38	7.9	7.47	7.09	6.74	6.43
165	2:20	14.48	13.22	12.17	11.26	10.49	9.81	9.22	8.69	8.22	7.8	7.42	7.07
175	2:15	15.36	14.03	12.9	11.95	11.12	10.41	9.78	9.22	8.72	8.27	7.87	7.5
200	2:10	17.55	16.03	14.75	13.65	12.71	11.89	11.17	10.53	9.96	9.45	8.99	8.57
220	2:07	19.31	17.63	16.22	15.02	13.98	13.08	12.29	11.59	10.96	10.4	9.89	9.43
240	2:05	21.07	19.24	17.7	16.39	15.26	14.27	13.41	12.64	11.96	11.34	10.79	10.29
250	2:00	21.94	20.03	18.43	17.07	15.89	14.86	13.96	13.16	12.45	11.81	11.24	10.72
260	1:58	22.82	20.84	19.17	17.75	16.52	15.46	14.52	13.69	12.95	12.29	11.69	11.14
275	1:55	24.14	22.04	20.28	18.78	17.48	16.35	15.36	14.48	13.7	13	12.37	11.79

*Row rate for 'Concept II' ergometers.

(J. Buckley, Lifestyle Fitness, Shrewsbury, 1996)

Table 7.5   METs conversion to walking pace

METs	kph	min/mile
2	2.3	approx. 40 min
3	3.4	approx. 31 min
4	4.5	23:30
5	5.6	17:40
6	6.8	14:54
7	7.9	12:50
8	9.0	10:45
9	10.2	9:29
10	11.3	8:20
11	12.4	7:48

Ensuring a clear understanding of the concept of exercise workrate

Chapters 4, 8 and 9 describe the direct relationship between workrate or speed (exercise intensity) and the demand for oxygen or oxygen consumption ($\dot{V}O_2$). Because heart rate and RPE are also directly related to $\dot{V}O_2$ (see Chapters 4 and 6), then when these are measured during an activity (e.g. exercise cycling) they represent a proportion (percentage) of that individual's maximum exercising capacity. It is therefore paramount that the exercise professional has an understanding of cycle ergometer intensities equivalent to other activities or household chores, not just from a prescriptive angle but also from a physiological demand perspective.

For example, a workrate of 60 W on an exercise cycle, which for most healthy active individuals seems fairly easy, may tax about 70% of an unhealthy or untrained individual's capacity and thus render them to fatigue in less than 10–12 minutes. If this is the case, they may find typical home chore activities quite demanding. A cycle workrate of 60 W performed by a man of 75 kg (165 lb or 11 stone 10 lb) is equivalent to walking at approximately 2.5–3 mph (4.1 kph; see Table 7.4) or mowing the lawn or moderate digging (see Table 7.2 and 7.3). The tables illustrate how valuable the relationship between heart rate, RPE and workrate is. It is important to understand, therefore, that what some people classify as easy work (e.g. easy gardening or a gentle stroll), others performing exactly the same activity at the same level may find very taxing and describe it as hard gardening or a very brisk walk. When recommending such activities (e.g. gardening), it is important to consider the energy requirements of activities, as outlined in the above tables. For more specific gymnasium exercise intensities, Chapter 9 describes the relationship between a person's $\dot{V}O_{2max}$ and workrate or speed on exercise cycles, rowing ergometers and motorized treadmills.

A typical case question

If a client (especially an older person) asks 'Is gardening and brisk walking good enough for me to improve my fitness?', you should be able to advise them, based on having carried out a very simple 5-minute cycle test between 50 and 70 W and seeing if they struggle, as determined by their effort. Is RPE > 13 or is their heart rate > 80% of maximum or > 80% of maximal heart rate reserve (Table 7.1.)? If RPE is above 13 or heart rate above 80% of maximum, you will know that they will probably find what most people consider easy gardening or steady walking as being quite hard. Your advice should certainly include making a statement about the level to which they should exert themselves. By approaching it from this perspective, not only do you as the exercise professional set a standardized assessment level, but the client will set their own standardized task (the gardening or the walk) as a means of self-assessment. Noticeable improvements in being able to perform everyday tasks are far more meaningful to a client than the exercise science results measured by the exercise professional.

If tasks have demanded more than 50% of a person's capacity (Chapter 1, Figure 1.3), then such activity is of an intensity to improve fitness, and thus the client's subjective benefits will be confirmed with your scientific measures showing improvement. If you were advising a sedentary client who felt 50–60 W of cycling was much easier (RPE < 11 or < 60% HR_{max}), then your advice about their gardening and walking performed regularly would be to say 'It may not confer any noticeable fitness benefit but certainly there are health benefits to your blood and circulation as well as psychological benefits'. *Prior to commencing such a test it is assumed that the person is healthy and able to exercise as determined by the family doctor.*

Establishing exercise workrates or target heart rates from ratings of perceived exertion during a submaximal exercise cycle test

At this point, possibly more than any other point in this book, the reader should ensure that they clearly understand the assessment protocol to follow. From the authors' experience, and in their opinion, this protocol and the related examples are the most versatile prescription tools to be described in the book.

The following protocol has the versatility to be used in the same way for all clients, whether they are an average healthy sedentary person wishing to become a little more active, an athletically inclined person, or even a cardiac patient. It is a protocol which takes into consideration whether or not the client's heart rate is atypically fast or if their heart rate is atypically slow or artifically slowed from medication (e.g. beta blockers). It accommodates for the possibility that even if a minor heart condition is present, where it is difficult to get an accurate heart rate during exercise, your client can be given a specified workrate that will be beneficial.

In Chapters 4 and 6 it was stated that during submaximal exercise there is a direct and linear relationship between exercise workrate, heart rate and RPE. What this means is that as exercise intensity increases there is a corresponding straight-line increase in either heart or RPE. If the client is on beta blocker medication, as will be shown in Chapter 11 and was briefly covered in Chapter 6 (Figure 6.10), this relationship holds true. The only difference is that the heart rate at any given workrate or RPE is decreased by a constant 20–40 beats per minute. It is from this relationship that it is possible, as will be demonstrated in Figures 7.6 and 7.7, to determine a person's beneficial individual exercise intensity, whether it be at a low level just for health gain or at higher levels for both health and fitness gains.

Much of the following protocol can be adapted for use with other ergometers (e.g. treadmills, rowers), so long as there is a measurement of workrate and the problems with skill and measuring heart rate, as mentioned earlier, are overcome. The protocol is as follows.

1. Ensure you have an exercise cycle ergometer that produces an accurate readout of both pedal speed (pedals or revolutions per minute; rpm) and watts (workrate). A high-quality cycle may be more important for your less fit, less active and possibly less well clients, who need to feel comfortable and easily in control of the cycle.
2. Set up a data sheet as in Figure 7.1(a) and set up blank graphs as in Figures 7.1(b,c) (have these blanks photocopied for multiple use, a copy for each client).
3. Ensure that a thorough health history screening procedure has been performed either by the exercise assessor or the family doctor; *better still, both!* (see Chapter 12).
4. Obtain a recent (past 2–6 months) activity or exercise training history from the client to determine how familiar they are with physical exertion.
5. Set up the exercise cycle so that the saddle height and handlebars are adjusted to the correct level.
6. Check that the heart rate monitoring system is working (possibly check it earlier on yourself both at rest and under exercise conditions).
7. Have the client sitting on the exercise cycle and describe the standardized use of the RPE scale as outlined in Chapter 6.
8. Explain that the aim is to get the client to cycle at a steady controllable pace for 6 minutes; if the initial intensity is set correctly, most clients will have no problem completing this task.
9. Most females will be comfortable at either a pedal speed of 50 or 60 rpm and males at 65–75 rpm; possibly use the first minute of the assessment to determine this, but afterwards ensure that they maintain a very constant rate (see Chapter 8, Table 8.1).
10. The initial resistance should be set to a relatively low level initially (see Chapter 8, Table 8.1), in order that the client can pedal comfortably and is able to ease into the assessment (e.g. for untrained sedentary individuals 25–40 W).
11. After 2 minutes of cycling, if the RPE is < 8 increase the workrate by 100% (i.e. from 25 to 50 W); if the RPE is 9 or 10 increase the workrate by about 50% (i.e. 40 to 60 W). For cardiac, high blood

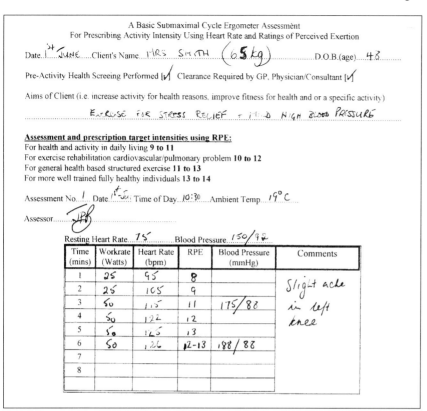

Figure 7.1 (a) A data sheet (Sample 1) for collecting heart rate and RPE data during submaximal cycle ergometry.

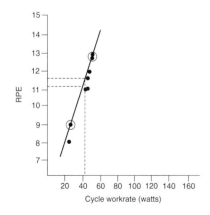

Figure 7.1 (b) A chart (Sample 1) for plotting RPE responses to given cycle workrates.

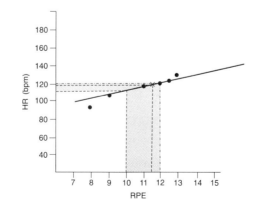

Figure 7.1 (c) A chart (Sample 1) for plotting heart rate responses to a given RPE.

A Basic Submaximal Cycle Ergometer Assessment
For Prescribing Activity Intensity Using Heart Rate and Ratings of Perceived Exertion

Date.................Client's Name...D.O.B.(age)..................

Pre-Activity Health Screeing Performed [ ]   Clearance Required by GP, Physician/Consultant [ ]

Aims of Client (i.e. increase activity for health reasons, improve fitness for health and or a specific activity)

....

Assessment and prescription target intensities using RPE:
For health and activity in daily living **9 to 11**
For exercise rehabilitation cardiovascular/pulmonary problem **10 to 12**
For general health based structured exercise **11 to 13**
For more well trained fully healthy individuals **13 to 14**

Assessment No...... Date........... Time of Day..............Ambient Temp.................

Assessor...............

Resting Heart Rate...................Blood Pressure....................

Time (mins)	Workrate (Watts)	Heart Rate (bpm)	RPE	Blood Pressure (mmHg)	Comments
1					
2					
3					
4					
5					
6					
7					
8					

pressure or elderly clients it may be desirable to start at even lower than 25 W.

12. It is important to remember that whenever the workrate is changed, at least 3 minutes is required to allow the new responses (heart rate and RPE) to rise and then level off. If the initial intensity is set too low, all this means is that the test may take a little longer (up to 7 or 8 minutes).

13. By the end of 6–8 minutes the aim is to have the RPE levelled off at 11–13 and then to determine either a target heart rate or workrates using Figure 7.1 (b,c) and Table 7.4.

Using the cycle workrate, heart rate and RPE data to approximate exercise intensity and or/establish a target heart rate

Two client samples have been produced using the data sheets of Figures 7.1(a) and 7.2(a) and the graphs in Figures 7.1(b,c) and 7.2(b,c). For information regarding the full consultation process see Chapter 12.

In Sample 1 and Figure 7.1(a), Mrs Smith has been recommended by her doctor either to be more active or possibly a little fitter to help with her borderline hypertension (blood pressure). She has recently moved house

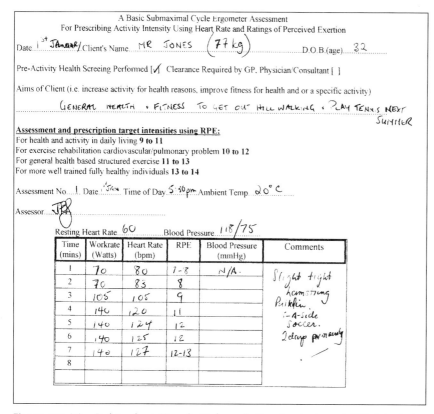

Figure 7.2 (a) A data sheet (Sample 2) for collecting heart rate and RPE data during submaximal cycle ergometry.

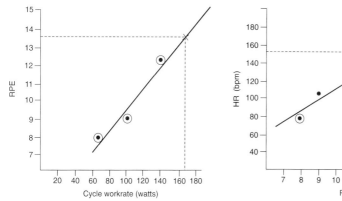

Figure 7.2 (b) A chart (Sample 2) for plotting RPE responses to given cycle workrates.

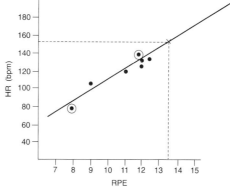

Figure 7.2 (c) A chart (Sample 2) for plotting heart rate responses to a given RPE.

A Basic Submaximal Cycle Ergometer Assessment
For Prescribing Activity Intensity Using Heart Rate and Ratings of Perceived Exertion

Date.................Client's Name...D.O.B.(age)...............

Pre-Activity Health Screeing Performed [ ]   Clearance Required by GP, Physician/Consultant [ ]

Aims of Client (i.e. increase activity for health reasons, improve fitness for health and or a specific activity)

....

Assessment and prescription target intensities using RPE:
For health and activity in daily living **9 to 11**
For exercise rehabilitation cardiovascular/pulmonary problem **10 to 12**
For general health based structured exercise **11 to 13**
For more well trained fully healthy individuals **13 to 14**

Assessment No....... Date........... Time of Day...............Ambient Temp................

Assessor...

Resting Heart Rate....................Blood Pressure................

Time (mins)	Workrate (Watts)	Heart Rate (bpm)	RPE	Blood Pressure (mmHg)	Comments
1					
2					
3					
4					
5					
6					
7					
8					

and has had to take on more responsibility at work due to her employer down-sizing the business. She has done little exercise for the past 15–20 years and stated that she was never good at games or sport at school and found cross-country running more difficult than most of her classmates.

She feels she can manage 40 minutes twice per week to attend the health club gym in town either during her lunch break or straight after work, and is willing to be more active around her home and village at weekends. When she comes to the gym she will have time to use the rowing machine and cycle and treadmill, but is concerned about using a stepping machine because of the slight ache (possible arthritis) in her left knee.

Method 1. Setting Mrs Smith's initial exercise intensity (approximately 55–60% of her aerobic capacity using RPE and cycle workrate)

In reviewing the data, the highest RPE given at each of the two workloads (25 and 50 W) were 9 and 13, respectively. These are circled in Figure 7.1(b). For her health and fitness needs, Mrs Smith should be working for her 40 minutes at a workrate which elicits an RPE between 10 and 12 and certainly no higher than 13, as stated earlier, and summarized in Figure 7.1(a).

In acknowledging the linear relationship between RPE, workrate and oxygen demand stated in Chapters 4 and 6, an individualized intensity of activity can be established for Mrs Smith. It is established by drawing a straight *trend line* between the highest RPE elicited at each workrate and then using the trend line to establish the cycle workrate which corresponds to the beneficial RPE range best suited to Mrs Smith's needs. The beneficial RPE range, considering her present minor cardio-vascular problem of high blood pressure, is 10–12. The trend line intersection of the horizontal dotted line of the RPE at 11 drops a vertical line down to approximately 40–50 W of cycle workrate.

Table 7.4 can be used to calculate treadmill and rowing ergometer intensities which are equivalent to 40–50 W on an exercise cycle. Mrs Smith's treadmill pace to start with will be around 4–4.5 kph, a rowing pace of about 3:40 (minutes:seconds) to cover each 500 m (500 m split-time). Including 5–7 minutes of warm-up time, Mrs Smith's 40-minute programme will thus include 30–35 minutes of activity divided between the cycle, rower and treadmill. After a few attendances at the gym, she could be given the option to adjust the timings on these pieces of equipment, spending longer on those machines she finds more suitable and less on those less desirable, but still totalling 30–35 minutes in all. Over time, however, her familiarity with exercise and her fitness will increase, typically making her want to work to higher intensities. This will be addressed in a later section on alteration and progression of programmes.

Method 2. Setting Mrs Smith's programme by a target heart rate

Even if Mrs Smith had arrived for her consultation having been put on beta blocker medication by her doctor, this method would still work. It would only be invalidated if at some point her medication dosage was changed or stopped. A simple re-evaluation, however, could quickly be done to re-establish a new target heart rate (see Chapter 11 for further considerations of people on cardiovascular medication).

In Figure 7.1(c), the target exercise heart rate is determined again from the intersection on the trend line of the heart rate response which corresponds to the RPE range of 10–12. The trend line is drawn as the best possible straight line through the middle of the data points from the lowest to the highest heart rate. From the graph it can be seen that this target heart rate is around 115–120 bpm. The prescription would be for Mrs Smith to adjust the intensities of the machines to maintain her heart rate, for the 30–35 minute programme, around 115–120 bpm. These intensities should thus be very similar to those prescribed in Method 1 above. Method 2 requires the use of an accurate heart rate monitoring system (monitoring systems are described in Chapter 6).

It must be stated that there is a key advantage of this method over the age-predicted maximal heart rate or heart rate reserve methods (see Chapter 6 and Table 7.1). Establishing heart rate by the RPE workload method is completely independent of variabilities of age and medication which are inherent in the age-predicted methods. This method is completely accommodating to the individual client, especially if they have an atypically fast or low pulse rate. It is obvious that this method may become more valid with older clients, as it was shown in Chapter 6 that the variability in age-predicted maximal heart rate increases with age.

Alteration and progression of a programme

Combining Method 1 and/or 2 and the RPE effort production method

Method 1 is one of the best ways to minimize the amount of guesswork or trial and error in the initial stages of getting someone started on an exercise programme (see Chapter 9 for other ways). With either the target heart or the RPE effort production method (described in Chapter 6) the client would initially have to try different workrates or speeds until they found an intensity which produced the required RPE or heart rate. If the client is inexperienced with the sensation of more vigorous activity, or it has been a long time since they last participated, there is the chance that they may initially select too high a pace. With too high a pace they may be confronted with a sense of failure from being unable to complete in the prescribed time.

Method 1 greatly increases the possibility of getting the right pace quickly. The client is then familiarized with their workrates and thereafter knows each time they attend or perform their activities they will be confident of sustaining the correct pace. But as stated in Method 1, a time comes when their fitness and/or confidence will allow them to perform at higher intensities and the programme must be progressed.

The RPE effort production and the RPE target heart rate methods automatically allow for progression to occur. As a person becomes fitter and more comfortable with their programme their physiological adaptations will require them to work harder in order to elicit the required RPE or target heart rate, as described in Chapters 4 and 5. Because of the great practical advantage RPE has over measuring heart rate, it tends to become the favoured tool. It is important to ensure that there are RPE scales on equipment, on the walls and near to all aerobic exercise equipment.

Name.. MRS SMITH

Aerobic Exercise Machines

Target RPE 10-12 ...... Target Heart Rate 115 - 120 bpm

Ergometer	1st JUNE	24th JUNE	24th JULY	
Cycle	12 mins 40-50 WATTS	55 WATTS	65-70 WATTS	
Treadmill	10 min 4-4.5kph	5kph	5-5.5 kph	
Rower	8 min 3:40/500	3:20/50	3:00/500	
Stepper	N/A KNEES ?	POSSIBLY TRY WHEN FITTER	TRY 2 mins at 150 WATTS	

Figure 7.3 Sample of an aerobic exercise programme card. Here, Mrs Smith, by 24th July, is making an equivalent effort to completing 1 mile in 18–20 minutes.

A good exercise prescription includes intensity settings, target heart rate and/or target RPE

It is recommended that the exercise prescription contains a prescribed workrate or intensity (i.e. watts, speed, etc.) in the very initial stages and then a target RPE and/or target heart rate for the future.

Figure 7.3 is an example of an exercise programme card which records the initial intensity along with the target RPE and heart rate. The target RPE and heart rate remain the same over time, but the workrate/intensities have been adjusted with increases in fitness.

The daily activity programme for Mrs Smith

One of the benefits of Mrs Smith attending a gym-based programme is that it allows her to 'learn' how to know what her beneficial physical limits are. When she then becomes active around the home or whenever she is 'on the move', she will be able to compare her sensations to those felt while working out in the gym. A pocket-sized RPE scale may be helpful and she knows that as long as she is at 9 or above she will be getting some health benefit (physically and psychologically) as long as she accumulates 30 minutes in at least 10-minute bouts over the course of the day.

So those clients who may even only visit the exercise centre once per week, but with a structured programme to the right intensity, will be able to answer if someone asks: 'what's the point of going to the gym if you don't really get any fitness gains?' That one session per week will:

- have some social and psychological benefit,
- establish a measure of intensity to which the client can compare their exertion sensations when performing activity in their daily life,
- act as a means of assessment if the client's home activity programme is vigorous enough to provide some fitness gain,
- lead to finding time to attend the gym more often. If a sense of achievment and enjoyment is gained, this may have further physical, psychological and social health benefits and help to sustain the 'process' of being physically active.

The above example links with the concept of stages of behavioural change in Chapter 3, where it is not necessarily the rate of change of behaviour which is the most important element, but the fact that change is occurring.

In Sample 2 (Figures 7.2a–c), it is clear there is a more established fitness focus to Mr Jones's programme, but which will certainly bring health gains too. The aim is to get this client working up to RPE levels of 14. The trend line method used is exactly the same as for Mrs Smith, in Sample 1, but resulting in an initial cycle workrate of 160–170 W and a target exercise heart rate of about 155 bpm. The equivalent intensities on the treadmill would be approximately 9–10 kph and 2:25/500 split time on the rowing ergometer (see Table 7.4b).

If Mr Jones wanted to do some running, the recommended pace converted from kilometres per hour to minutes per mile would be 9:30 to 10:00 minutes per mile (see Chapter 9, Table 9.2). He should thus be able to complete 3 miles (5 km) in about 30 minutes. Regular training at these levels of intensity of a few months will certainly help with the tennis and hill walking (hiking) he has planned for the summer. As the better weather approaches he may find he wishes to use the gym less, but this should not make gym training redundant. The gym programme allows for him to alter and progress his pace based on his target RPE or heart rate, from which then he can re-establish his outdoor running pace as he becomes fitter. He may wish to do more work on muscular strength and flexibility when he comes to the gym and leave a greater proportion of his aerobic training to the outdoor activities, assuming he his working to the correct intensities.

The exercise professional who is confident in applying the material in this book should most certainly be able to assist in the programme progression of people like Mrs Smith and Mr Jones, exampled above.

Chapter summary

From an activity and exercise programming perspective this chapter may be the most valuable part of this book. By now the reader should have a clear understanding of the differences between health achieved through increased daily activity and health and fitness gains from more structured and more vigorous activity and exercise. This chapter is closely linked with Chapters 1 and 2 and aims to give the exercise or health professional the means of playing a key role in tackling the growing problem of the sedentary Western society lifestyle. Finally, the concepts of this chapter are versatile enough to be used on a wide range of clients, from people wanting to lose weight and reduce blood pressure to those wanting to truly improve fitness for health and other leisure pursuits.

References

1. Karvonen, M., Kentala, A. and Mustala, O. (1957) The effects of training on heart rate: a longitudinal study. *Ann. Med. Biol. Fenn.*, **35**, 307–315.
2. Ainsworth, B.E., Haskell, W.L., Leon, A.S. *et al.* (1993) Compendium of physical activities. *Med. Sci. Sports Exec.*, **25**, 71–80.

8

Protocols for predicting and estimating aerobic capacity

Review of the protocols
Considerations for choosing the appropriate predictive $\dot{V}O_{2max}$
protocol
References

For at least four decades researchers have been developing protocols for predicting maximal aerobic capacity ($\dot{V}O_{2max}$). The objectives for doing so have ranged from minimizing the various complexities, time and costs involved in direct laboratory measurements of $\dot{V}O_{2max}$ to providing valid fitness tests that can be conducted in safety in the field. One of the most notable protocols is the exercise cycle test using the Astrand–Ryhming nomogram which was developed in 1954.[1] This protocol and many that have followed[2–9] are based either upon heart rate response and/or a distance/time performance score in relation to a predetermined bout of exercise (e.g. cycle ergometry, walking, running, step-ups, ergometer rowing).

With any predictive measure of $\dot{V}O_{2max}$, criticism of validity is inevitable. A number of the protocols, such as the Astrand cycle test, the Chester step test and the Canadian standardized test of fitness, have however received continued attention to increase their validity. For the purposes of this book it is assumed that the various protocols are reasonable predictors, that the research behind them is robust and that they are valuable tools for allowing individuals to be assessed outside of the standard modern exercise physiology laboratory.

Review of the protocols

The protocols to be reviewed include tests which can be performed from guidelines in this chapter:

- the Astrand submaximal cycle test,[1,10]
- the Rockport 1-mile walk test,[2]
- Cooper's 12-minute run field test,[*3]
- the McArdle step test,[4]

- the Keele Lifestyle nomogram for predicting $\dot{V}O_{2max}$ from ratings of perceived exertion,[11]

and tests which require the purchase of a package from a sports governing body or equipment manufacturer:

- the Canadian standardized test of fitness step test,[5]
- the British National Coaching Foundation (NCF) multi-stage fitness test,[*6,7]
- the Concept II rowing ergometer test for predicting $\dot{V}O_{2max}$,[*8]
- the Chester step test.[9]

This is by no means a complete list of protocols which have been developed. Those tests marked by an asterisk may require near to maximal effort and are not suitable for untrained/non-athletic clients or for those who are over the age of 35 years.

It is paramount, as will be described in Chapter 12, that a general resting health screening assessment/medical history or medical examination is performed prior to carrying out any of the following protocols.

The Astrand submaximal cycle ergometer test

The test is performed for 6 minutes on a standard cycle ergometer (e.g. Monark) on which workrate, in watts, can accurately be measured. It requires an accurate measure of heart rate taken at the end of each minute. The aim is to raise the subject's heart rate to at least 120 beats per minute (bpm) within the first 2 minutes of cycling. If this is not achieved, the workload should be increased by 50% for untrained and 100% for trained or young subjects, respectively. Table 8.1 provides a guide to choosing appropriate starting pedal speeds and workrates.

If the workload has to be increased during the test, at least 3 minutes should be allowed for the heart rate to plateau in relation to the workrate. The average heart rate of the 5th and 6th minute is required for the calculation of $\dot{V}O_{2max}$. However, if the difference in heart rates between these two intervals is more than 5 bpm, the test should be continued until the steady state is reached. The heart rate should not exceed 200 minus the subject's age unless previous medical clearance is given of an atypical fast heart rate (tachycardia). If the heart rate does

Table 8.1 Recommended starting pedal speeds and workrates for the Astrand submaximal cycle ergometer test

Training status	Males		Females	
	Pedal speed (rpm)	Workrate (Watts)	Pedal speed (rpm)	Workrate (W)
Sedentary or age 50+	60	30–50	50–60	25–30
Moderately active	70	70	60	60
Highly active/trained	75–85	75–85	60–75	60–75

reach this level, the test should be stopped and this heart rate noted, with related comments, and used as the value for the calculation of $\dot{V}O_{2max}$. In such atypical cases the predicted $\dot{V}O_{2max}$ may possibly be underestimated and use of a RPE[12] may be helpful. Monitoring blood pressure during the test of subjects with atypical tachycardias is useful, where the systolic pressure should rise with each workrate increase but where diastolic pressure either increases or decreases slightly (no more than $\pm 5\,mmHg$).

Using the Astrand–Ryhming nomogram to predict $\dot{V}O_{2max}$

From Tables 8.2(a) (for males) and 8.2(b) (for females) adopt the following procedure:

1. Find the heart rate in the left-hand column which is nearest to the average from the 5th and 6th minute of the test.
2. Read across to the column of the workrate which was being performed at the end of the test.

Table 8.2 (a)   Method for predicting $\dot{V}O_{2max}$ during submaximal exercise cycling. (Adapted from the Astrand–Ryhming nomogram)

MALES

WR: HR	50	55	60	65	70	75	80	90	100	105	110	120	130	140	150
120	2.2	2.3	2.4	2.6	2.7	2.8	3	3.2	3.5	3.6	3.7	4	4.2	4.5	4.8
122	2.1	2.2	2.3	2.5	2.6	2.7	2.8	3.1	3.4	3.5	3.6	3.9	4.1	4.4	4.7
124	2	2.15	2.35	2.4	2.5	2.65	2.75	3	3.3	3.4	3.5	3.7	4	4.2	4.5
126	1.95	2.1	2.25	2.35	2.45	2.6	2.7	2.9	3.2	3.6	3.4	3.65	3.85	4.1	4.4
128	1.9	2.05	2.15	2.3	2.4	2.5	2.65	2.8	3.15	3.2	3.3	3.5	3.75	4	4.2
130	1.85	2	2.1	2.2	2.35	2.4	2.6	2.75	3	3.1	3.2	3.4	3.6	3.9	4.1
132	1.8	1.95	2.05	2.15	2.3	2.35	2.5	2.7	2.9	3	3.1	3.3	3.5	3.75	4
134	1.75	1.9	2	2.1	2.2	2.3	2.4	2.65	2.8	2.9	3	3.2	3.4	3.65	3.9
136	1.7	1.85	1.95	2.05	2.15	2.2	2.35	2.6	2.75	2.8	2.95	3.15	3.35	3.6	3.8
138	1.65	1.8	1.9	2	2.1	2.15	2.3	2.5	2.7	2.75	2.9	3.1	3.25	3.5	3.7
140	1.6	1.75	1.8	1.95	2.05	2.1	2.2	2.4	2.6	2.7	2.8	3	3.2	3.4	3.6
142	1.58	1.7	1.75	1.9	2	2.01	2.15	2.35	2.55	2.65	2.75	2.9	3.1	3.3	3.5
144	1.5	1.65	1.7	1.85	1.95	2	2.1	2.3	2.5	2.6	2.7	2.85	3	3.25	3.4
146		1.6	1.65	1.8	1.9	1.95	2.05	2.25	2.4	2.55	2.6	2.8	2.95	3.15	3.3
148			1.6	1.75	1.85	1.9	2	2.2	2.35	2.5	2.55	2.75	2.9	3.1	3.25
150				1.7	1.8	1.85	1.95	2.15	2.3	2.4	2.5	2.7	2.8	3	3.2
152				1.65	1.75	1.8	1.9	2.1	2.25	2.35	2.45	2.65	2.75	2.95	3.1
154				1.6	1.7	1.8	1.85	2.05	2.2	2.3	2.4	2.6	2.7	2.9	3
156					1.65	1.75	1.8	2	2.15	2.25	2.3	2.6	2.65	2.8	2.95
158						1.6	1.7	1.75	1.95	2.1	2.2	2.25	2.5	2.6	2.75	2.9
160						1.55	1.65	1.7	1.9	2.1	2.15	2.2	2.45	2.55	2.7	2.85
162							1.6	1.7	1.85	2.05	2.1	2.2	2.35	2.5	2.65	2.8
164								1.65	1.8	2	2.05	2.15	2.3	2.45	2.6	2.75
166								1.6	1.8	1.95	2	2.1	2.25	2.4	2.55	2.7
168									1.75	1.9	2	2.05	2.2	2.35	2.5	2.65
170									1.7	1.85	1.95	2	2.15	2.3	2.45	2.6

WR = workrate (Watts); HR = heart rate (bpm).

Table 8.2 (b)   Method for predicting $\dot{V}O_{2max}$ during submaximal exercise cycling. (Adapted from the Astrand–Ryhming nomogram)

FEMALES

WR: HR	50	55	60	65	70	75	80	90	100	105	110	120	130
120	2.5	2.6	2.8	2.9	3.1	3.2	3.4	3.7	4.1	4.2	4.4	4.6	5
122	2.4	2.5	2.7	2.8	3	3.1	3.3	3.6	3.9	4.1	4.2	4.4	4.8
124	2.3	2.4	2.6	2.7	2.9	3	3.2	3.4	3.8	3.9	4.1	4.2	4.6
126	2.2	2.3	2.5	2.6	2.8	2.9	3	3.3	3.6	3.7	3.9	4.1	4.4
128	2.15	2.25	2.4	2.5	2.7	2.75	2.9	3.2	3.5	3.6	3.7	4	4.3
130	2.05	2.2	2.3	2.4	2.6	2.7	2.8	3.1	3.3	3.5	3.6	3.8	4.3
132	2	2.1	2.2	2.35	2.5	2.65	2.7	3	3.2	3.4	3.5	3.7	4
134	1.95	2.05	2.15	2.3	2.4	2.6	2.65	2.9	3.1	3.3	3.4	3.6	3.9
136	1.9	2	2.1	2.2	2.35	2.5	2.6	2.8	3	3.2	3.3	3.5	3.8
138	1.8	1.95	2	2.15	2.3	2.4	2.5	2.75	2.9	3.1	3.2	3.4	3.6
140	1.75	1.9	1.95	2.1	2.2	2.3	2.4	2.65	2.8	3	3.1	3.3	3.5
142	1.7	1.8	1.9	2.05	2.15	2.25	2.35	2.6	2.75	2.9	3	3.2	3.45
144	1.65	1.75	1.85	2	2.1	2.2	2.3	2.5	2.7	2.8	2.9	3.1	3.35
146	1.6	1.7	1.8	1.95	2.05	2.15	2.2	2.4	2.65	2.75	2.8	3	3.25
148	1.55	1.65	1.75	1.9	2	2.1	2.15	2.35	2.6	2.7	2.75	2.95	3.2
150	1.5	1.6	1.7	1.85	1.95	2.05	2.1	2.3	2.55	2.6	2.7	2.9	3.1
152		1.55	1.65	1.8	1.9	2	2.05	2.25	2.45	2.55	2.65	2.8	3
154		1.5	1.6	1.75	1.85	1.95	2	2.2	2.4	2.5	2.6	2.75	2.95
156			1.55	1.7	1.8	1.9	1.95	2.15	2.35	2.4	2.55	2.7	2.9
158			1.5	1.65	1.75	1.85	1.9	2.1	2.3	2.35	2.45	2.65	2.8
160				1.6	1.7	1.8	1.85	2.05	2.25	2.3	2.4	2.6	2.75
162					1.65	1.75	1.8	2	2.2	2.25	2.35	2.5	2.7
164					1.6	1.7	1.75	1.95	2.15	2.2	2.3	2.45	2.65
166						1.65	1.7	1.9	2.1	2.15	2.25	2.4	2.6
168						1.6	1.7	1.85	2.05	2.1	2.2	2.35	2.55
170						1.55	1.65	1.8	2	2.05	2.15	2.3	2.5

WR = workrate (Watts); HR = heart rate (bpm).

3. The value at this intersection is the predicted $\dot{V}O_{2max}$ (litres min^{-1}) uncorrected for age.
4. Use Table 8.3 to correct for age by reading down the left-hand column to the $\dot{V}O_{2max}$ estimated from the nomogram and then across to the appropriate age column (for ages 20–25 no correction for age is required).

To describe $\dot{V}O_{2max}$ in relation to body mass, which is necessary for prescribing weight-bearing activities or comparing individuals of different sizes, it is necessary to convert the score by either using the equation below as given in Chapter 4, or more quickly by using Table 8.4. From this table find the client's body weight (lb) or mass (kg) down the left-hand column, then read across the top row to their $\dot{V}O_{2max}$ in litres min^{-1}. The intersection of body mass and $\dot{V}O_{2max}$ gives the $\dot{V}O_{2max}$ in ml kg^{-1} min^{-1}.

$$\dot{V}O_{2max} \text{ [litres. } min^{-1} \times 1000 \text{ ml. } l^{-1} \div \text{ Body mass (kg)]}$$

$$= \dot{V}O_{2max} \text{ (ml. } kg^{-1}. min^{-1}) \text{ (see Table 8.4)}$$

Table 8.3   Age correction for oxygen uptake. (Adapted from Astrand and Rodahl[10])

Age: 25	15	35	40	45	50	55	60	65
1.5	1.6	1.3	1.2	1.2	1.1	1.1	1.0	1.0
1.6	1.8	1.4	1.3	1.2	1.2	1.1	1.1	1.0
1.7	1.9	1.5	1.4	1.3	1.3	1.2	1.2	1.1
1.8	2.0	1.6	1.5	1.4	1.4	1.3	1.2	1.2
1.9	2.1	1.7	1.6	1.5	1.4	1.4	1.3	1.2
2.0	2.2	1.7	1.6	1.6	1.5	1.4	1.4	1.3
2.1	2.3	1.8	1.7	1.6	1.6	1.5	1.4	1.4
2.2	2.4	1.9	1.8	1.7	1.7	1.6	1.5	1.4
2.3	2.5	2.0	1.9	1.8	1.7	1.6	1.6	1.5
2.4	2.6	2.1	2.0	1.9	1.8	1.7	1.6	1.6
2.5	2.8	2.2	2.1	2.0	1.9	1.8	1.7	1.6
2.6	2.9	2.3	2.2	2.0	2.0	1.8	1.8	1.7
2.7	3.0	2.4	2.2	2.1	2.0	1.9	1.8	1.8
2.8	3.1	2.4	2.3	2.2	2.1	2.0	1.9	1.8
2.9	3.2	2.5	2.4	2.3	2.2	2.1	2.0	1.9
3.0	3.3	2.6	2.5	2.3	2.3	2.1	2.0	2.0
3.1	3.4	2.7	2.6	2.4	2.3	2.2	2.1	2.0
3.2	3.5	2.8	2.7	2.5	2.4	2.3	2.2	2.1
3.3	3.6	2.9	2.7	2.6	2.5	2.3	2.2	2.1
3.4	3.7	3.0	2.8	2.7	2.6	2.4	2.3	2.2
3.5	3.9	3.0	2.9	2.7	2.6	2.5	2.4	2.3
3.6	4.0	3.1	3.0	2.8	2.7	2.6	2.5	2.3
3.7	4.1	3.2	3.1	2.9	2.8	2.6	2.5	2.4
3.8	4.2	3.3	3.2	3.0	2.9	2.7	2.6	2.5
3.9	4.3	3.4	3.2	3.0	2.9	2.8	2.7	2.5
4.0	4.4	3.5	3.3	3.1	3.0	2.8	2.7	2.6
4.1	4.5	3.6	3.4	3.2	3.1	2.9	2.8	2.7
4.2	4.6	3.7	3.5	3.3	3.2	3.0	2.9	2.7
4.3	4.7	3.7	3.6	3.4	3.2	3.1	2.9	2.8
4.4	4.8	3.8	3.7	3.4	3.3	3.1	3.0	2.9
4.5	4.9	3.9	3.7	3.5	3.4	3.2	3.1	2.9
4.6	5.1	4.0	3.8	3.6	3.5	3.3	3.1	3.0
4.7	5.2	4.1	3.9	3.7	3.5	3.3	3.2	3.1
4.8	5.3	4.2	4.0	3.7	3.6	3.4	3.3	3.1
4.9	5.4	4.3	4.1	3.8	3.7	3.5	3.3	3.2
5.0	5.5	4.3	4.2	3.9	3.8	3.6	3.4	3.3
5.1	5.6	4.4	4.2	4.0	3.8	3.6	3.5	3.3
5.2	5.7	4.5	4.3	4.1	3.9	3.7	3.5	3.4
5.3	5.8	4.6	4.4	4.1	4.0	3.8	3.6	3.4
5.4	5.9	4.7	4.5	4.2	4.1	3.8	3.7	3.5
5.5	6.0	4.8	4.6	4.3	4.1	3.9	3.7	3.6
5.6	6.2	4.9	4.6	4.4	4.2	4.0	3.8	3.6
5.7	6.3	5.0	4.7	4.4	4.3	4.0	3.9	3.7
5.8	6.4	5.0	4.8	4.5	4.4	4.1	4.0	3.8
5.9	6.5	5.1	4.9	4.6	4.4	4.2	4.0	3.8
6.0	6.6	5.2	5.0	4.7	4.5	4.3	4.1	3.9

The row label (rotated, left side): Result from the nomogram (litres. min^{-1})

Table 8.4 Conversion table of $\dot{V}O_{2max}$ from litres. min^{-1} to ml. kg^{-1} min^{-1}

Body Weight (lb)	(kg)	Maximal oxygen uptake (litres min^{-1})																						
		1.5	1.6	1.7	1.8	1.9	2.0	2.1	2.2	2.3	2.4	2.5	2.6	2.7	2.8	2.9	3.0	3.1	3.2	3.3	3.4	3.5	3.6	3.7	3.8
110	50	30	32	34	36	38	40	42	44	46	48	50	52	54	56	58	60	62	64	66	68	70	72	74	76
112	51	29	31	33	35	37	39	41	43	45	47	49	51	53	55	57	59	61	63	65	67	69	71	73	75
115	52	29	31	33	35	37	38	40	42	44	46	48	50	52	54	56	58	60	62	63	65	67	69	71	73
117	53	28	30	32	34	36	38	40	42	43	45	47	49	51	53	55	57	58	60	62	64	66	68	70	72
119	54	28	30	31	33	35	37	39	41	43	44	46	48	50	52	54	56	57	59	61	63	65	67	69	70
121	55	27	29	31	33	35	36	38	40	42	44	45	47	49	51	53	55	56	58	60	62	64	65	67	69
123	56	27	29	30	32	34	36	38	39	41	43	45	46	48	50	52	54	55	57	59	61	63	64	66	68
126	57	26	28	30	32	33	35	37	39	40	42	44	46	47	49	51	53	54	56	58	60	61	63	65	67
128	58	26	28	29	31	33	34	36	38	40	41	43	45	47	48	50	52	53	55	57	58	60	62	64	66
130	59	25	27	29	31	32	34	36	37	39	41	42	44	46	47	49	51	53	54	56	57	59	61	63	64
132	60	25	27	28	30	32	33	35	37	38	40	42	43	45	47	48	50	52	53	55	57	58	60	62	63
134	61	25	26	28	30	31	33	34	36	38	39	41	43	44	46	48	49	51	52	54	56	57	59	61	62
137	62	24	26	27	29	31	32	34	35	37	39	40	42	44	45	47	48	50	52	53	55	56	58	60	61
139	63	24	25	27	29	30	32	33	35	37	38	40	41	43	44	46	48	49	51	52	54	56	57	59	60
141	64	23	25	27	28	30	31	33	34	36	38	39	41	42	44	45	47	48	50	52	53	55	56	58	59
143	65	23	25	26	28	29	31	32	34	35	37	38	40	42	43	45	46	48	49	51	52	54	55	57	58
146	66	23	24	26	27	29	30	32	33	35	36	38	39	41	42	44	45	47	48	50	52	53	55	56	58
148	67	22	24	25	27	28	30	31	33	34	36	37	39	40	42	43	45	46	48	49	51	52	54	55	57
150	68	22	24	25	26	28	29	31	32	34	35	37	38	40	41	43	44	46	47	49	50	51	53	54	56
152	69	22	23	25	26	28	29	30	32	33	35	36	38	39	41	42	43	45	46	48	49	51	52	54	55
154	70	21	23	24	26	27	29	30	31	33	34	36	37	39	40	41	43	44	46	47	49	50	51	53	54
157	71	21	23	24	25	27	28	30	31	32	34	35	37	38	39	41	42	44	45	46	48	49	51	52	54
159	72	21	22	24	25	26	28	29	31	32	33	35	36	38	39	40	42	43	44	46	47	49	50	51	53
161	73	21	22	23	25	26	27	29	30	32	33	34	36	37	38	40	41	42	44	45	47	48	49	51	52
163	74	20	22	23	24	26	27	28	30	31	32	34	35	36	38	39	41	42	43	45	46	47	49	50	51
165	75	20	21	23	24	25	27	28	29	31	32	33	35	36	37	39	40	41	43	44	45	47	48	49	51
168	76	20	21	22	24	25	26	28	29	30	32	33	34	36	37	38	39	41	42	43	45	46	47	49	50
170	77	19	21	22	23	25	26	27	29	30	31	32	34	35	36	38	39	40	42	43	44	45	47	48	49
172	78	19	21	22	23	24	26	27	28	29	31	32	33	35	36	37	38	40	41	42	44	45	46	47	49
174	79	19	20	22	23	24	25	27	28	29	30	32	33	34	35	37	38	39	41	42	43	44	46	47	48
176	80	19	20	21	23	24	25	26	28	29	30	31	33	34	35	36	38	39	40	41	43	44	45	46	48
179	81	19	20	21	22	23	25	26	27	28	30	31	32	33	35	36	37	38	39	40	41	43	44	46	47
181	82	18	20	21	22	23	24	26	27	28	29	30	32	33	34	35	37	38	39	40	41	43	44	45	46
183	83	18	19	20	22	23	24	25	27	28	29	30	31	33	34	35	36	37	39	40	41	42	43	45	46
185	84	18	19	20	21	23	24	25	26	27	29	30	31	32	33	35	36	37	38	39	40	42	43	44	45
187	85	18	19	20	21	22	24	25	26	27	28	29	31	32	33	34	35	36	38	39	40	41	42	44	45
190	86	17	19	20	21	22	23	24	26	27	28	29	30	31	33	34	35	36	37	38	40	41	42	43	44
192	87	17	18	20	21	22	23	24	25	26	28	29	30	31	32	33	34	36	37	38	39	40	41	43	44
194	88	17	18	19	20	22	23	24	25	26	27	28	30	31	32	33	34	35	36	38	39	40	41	42	43
196	89	17	18	19	20	21	22	24	25	26	27	28	29	30	31	33	34	35	36	37	38	39	40	42	43
198	90	17	18	19	20	21	22	23	24	26	27	28	29	30	31	32	33	34	36	37	38	39	40	41	42
201	91	16	18	19	20	21	22	23	24	25	26	27	29	30	31	32	33	34	35	36	37	38	40	41	42
203	92	16	17	18	20	21	22	23	24	25	26	27	28	29	30	32	33	34	35	36	37	38	39	40	41
205	93	16	17	18	19	20	22	23	24	25	26	27	28	29	30	31	32	33	34	35	37	38	39	40	41
207	94	16	17	18	19	20	21	22	23	24	26	27	28	29	30	31	32	33	34	35	36	37	38	39	40
209	95	16	17	18	19	20	21	22	23	24	25	26	27	28	29	31	32	33	34	35	36	37	38	39	40
212	96	16	17	18	19	20	21	22	23	24	25	26	27	28	29	30	31	32	33	34	35	36	38	39	40
214	97	15	16	18	19	20	21	22	23	24	25	26	27	28	29	30	31	32	33	34	35	36	37	38	39
216	98	15	16	17	18	19	20	21	22	23	24	26	27	28	29	30	31	32	33	34	35	36	37	38	39
218	99	15	16	17	18	19	20	21	22	23	24	25	26	27	28	29	30	31	32	33	34	35	36	37	38
220	100	15	16	17	18	19	20	21	22	23	24	25	26	27	28	29	30	31	32	33	34	35	36	37	38

To use this table, read down the left-hand column to weight category and then across to the appropriate column of the clients $\dot{V}O_{2max}$ in litres per minute.

3.9	4.0	4.1	4.2	4.3	4.4	4.5	4.6	4.7	4.8	4.9	5.0	5.1	5.2	5.3	5.4	5.5	5.6	57	5.8	5.9	6.0
78	80	82	84	86	88	90	92	94	96	98	100	102	104	106	108	110	112	114	116	118	120
76	78	80	82	84	86	88	90	92	94	96	98	100	102	104	106	108	110	112	114	116	118
75	77	79	81	83	85	87	88	90	92	94	96	98	100	102	104	106	108	110	112	113	115
74	75	77	79	81	83	85	87	89	91	92	94	96	98	100	102	104	106	108	109	111	113
72	74	76	78	80	81	83	85	87	89	91	93	94	96	98	100	102	104	106	107	109	111
71	73	75	76	78	80	82	84	85	87	89	91	93	95	96	98	100	102	103	105	107	109
70	71	73	75	77	79	80	82	84	86	88	89	91	93	95	96	98	100	102	104	105	107
68	70	72	74	75	77	79	81	82	84	86	88	89	91	93	95	96	98	100	102	104	105
67	69	71	72	74	76	78	79	81	83	84	86	88	90	91	93	95	97	98	100	102	103
66	68	69	71	73	75	76	78	80	81	83	85	86	88	90	92	93	95	97	98	100	102
65	67	68	70	72	73	75	77	78	80	82	83	85	87	88	90	92	93	95	97	98	100
64	66	67	69	70	72	74	75	77	79	80	82	84	85	87	89	90	92	93	95	97	98
63	65	66	68	69	71	73	74	76	77	79	81	82	84	85	87	89	90	92	94	95	97
62	63	65	67	68	70	71	73	75	76	78	79	81	83	84	86	87	89	90	92	94	95
61	63	64	66	67	69	70	72	73	75	77	78	80	81	83	84	86	88	89	91	92	94
60	62	63	65	66	68	69	71	72	74	75	77	78	80	82	83	85	86	88	89	91	92
59	61	62	64	65	67	68	70	71	73	74	76	77	79	80	82	83	85	86	88	89	91
58	60	61	63	64	66	67	69	70	72	73	75	76	78	79	81	82	84	85	87	88	90
57	59	60	62	63	65	66	68	69	71	72	74	75	76	78	79	81	82	84	85	87	88
57	58	59	61	62	64	65	67	68	70	71	72	74	75	77	78	80	81	83	84	86	87
56	57	59	60	61	63	64	66	67	69	70	71	73	74	76	77	79	80	81	83	84	86
55	56	58	59	61	62	63	65	66	68	69	70	72	73	75	76	77	79	80	82	83	85
54	56	57	58	60	61	63	64	65	67	68	69	71	72	74	75	76	78	79	81	82	83
53	55	56	58	59	60	62	63	64	66	67	68	70	71	73	74	75	77	78	79	81	82
53	54	55	57	58	59	61	62	64	65	66	68	69	70	72	73	74	76	77	78	80	81
52	53	55	56	57	59	60	61	63	64	65	67	68	69	71	72	73	75	76	77	79	80
51	53	54	55	57	58	59	61	62	63	64	66	67	68	70	71	72	74	75	76	78	79
51	52	53	55	56	57	58	60	61	62	64	65	66	68	69	70	71	73	74	75	77	79
50	51	53	54	55	56	58	59	60	62	63	64	65	67	68	69	71	72	73	74	75	77
49	51	52	53	54	56	57	58	59	61	62	63	65	66	67	68	70	71	72	73	75	76
49	50	51	53	54	55	56	58	59	60	61	63	64	65	66	68	69	70	71	72	74	75
48	49	51	52	53	54	56	57	58	59	60	62	63	64	65	67	68	69	70	72	73	74
48	49	50	51	52	54	55	56	57	59	60	61	62	63	65	66	67	68	70	71	72	73
47	48	49	51	52	53	54	55	57	58	59	60	61	63	64	65	66	67	69	70	71	72
46	48	49	50	51	52	54	55	56	57	58	60	61	62	63	64	65	67	68	69	70	71
46	47	48	49	51	52	53	54	55	56	58	59	60	61	62	64	65	66	67	68	69	71
45	47	48	49	50	51	52	53	55	56	57	58	59	60	62	63	64	65	66	67	69	70
45	46	47	48	49	51	52	53	54	55	56	57	59	60	61	62	63	64	66	67	68	69
44	45	47	48	49	50	51	52	53	55	56	57	58	59	60	61	63	64	65	66	67	68
44	45	46	47	48	49	51	52	53	54	55	56	57	58	60	61	62	63	64	65	66	67
43	44	46	47	48	49	50	51	52	53	54	56	57	58	59	60	61	62	63	64	66	67
43	44	45	46	47	48	49	51	52	53	54	55	56	57	58	59	60	62	63	64	65	66
42	43	45	46	47	48	49	50	51	52	53	54	55	57	58	59	60	61	62	63	64	65
42	43	44	45	46	47	48	49	51	52	53	54	55	56	57	58	59	60	61	62	63	65
41	43	44	45	46	47	48	49	50	51	52	53	54	55	56	57	59	60	61	62	63	64
41	42	43	44	45	46	47	48	49	51	52	53	54	55	56	57	58	59	60	61	62	63
41	42	43	44	45	46	47	48	49	50	51	52	53	54	55	56	57	58	59	60	61	63
40	41	42	43	44	45	46	47	48	49	51	52	53	54	55	56	57	58	59	60	61	62
40	41	42	43	44	45	46	47	48	49	50	51	52	53	54	55	56	57	58	59	60	61
39	40	41	42	43	44	45	46	47	48	49	51	52	53	54	55	56	57	58	59	60	61
39	40	41	42	43	44	45	46	47	48	49	50	51	52	53	54	55	56	57	58	59	60

The Keele Lifestyle nomogram for predicting V̇O₂ₘₐₓ from ratings of perceived exertion (RPE)

There are some instances where predicting $\dot{V}O_{2max}$ using heart rate is neither possible nor valid, including:

- testing *an older individual* who may feel that they are working hard, yet their heart rate does not rise above 120 bpm, which makes using the Astrand or McArdle step test protocols invalid,
- testing an individual who has an *atypically fast or erratic pulse rate* from either a previously known condition or due to environmental or emotional factors,
- testing an individual who is on *medication* (e.g. beta blockers) that either slows down or speeds up the heart rate, which alters the typical response to exercise.

The Keele Lifestyle nomogram for predicting $\dot{V}O_{2max}$ from RPE follows the exact same protocol as the Astrand test above, except that RPE should not exceed a value of 15 at any time during the test. Ensure that the client has been properly instructed on standardized procedure for using the 15-point RPE scale, as outlined in Chapter 6. At the end of the 6-minute test, simply read down the left-hand column of Table 8.5 to the RPE given by the client in the 6th minute and then read across to the column of the workrate in watts.

The value of $\dot{V}O_{2max}$ is given in litres min^{-1}, which if necessary can be converted into ml kg^{-1} min^{-1} using Table 8.4.

The Rockport I-mile walk test

1. A 1-mile flat course is set out accurately (preferably on a track).
2. The course is marked off at quarter-mile intervals.
3. Subjects are asked to walk the mile course continuously and as fast as possible.
4. Heart rate is monitored continuously (recommended chest belt wireless transmitter and watch receiver monitor) and recorded at each quarter mile.
5. The overall time to complete the 1-mile walk is recorded.
6. $\dot{V}O_{2max}$ is predicted from the regression equation of Kline *et al.*[2]:

$$\dot{V}O_{2max} \text{ (litres min}^{-1}) = 6.9652 + (0.0091 \times Wt) - (0.0257 \times Age)$$
$$+ (0.5955 \times Sex) - (0.2240 \times T_1)$$
$$- (0.0115 \times AvHR_{1/4})$$

where Wt = body mass in lbs; sex = 1 for males, 0 for females; T_1 = time taken to complete 1-mile walk; and AvHR = Average of heart rates by summing recordings of each $\frac{1}{4}$ mile and dividing by 4.

Table 8.5　The Keele Lifestyle nomogram for predicting $\dot{V}O_{2max}$ from RPE during submaximal ergometer cycling. (From Buckley et al.[11], with permission)

RPE	$\dot{V}O_{2max}$	Cycle workrate (Watts)																				
		30	40	50	55	60	65	70	75	80	85	90	100	105	110	120	130	140	150	160	170	180
9	0.5	1.01	1.3	1.62	1.76	1.91	2.08	2.23	2.37	2.54	2.69	2.83	3.15	3.3	3.44	3.76	4.05	4.37	4.68	4.97	5.29	5.58
10	0.55	0.92	1.2	1.48	1.62	1.75	1.89	2.03	2.17	2.31	2.45	2.59	2.87	3.01	3.15	3.42	3.7	3.98	4.26	4.54	4.81	5.09
11	0.6	0.84	1.1	1.36	1.49	1.62	1.74	1.87	2	2.13	2.25	2.37	2.63	2.76	2.89	3.15	3.4	3.65	3.9	4.16	4.42	4.68
12	0.65	0.79	1.03	1.26	1.38	1.5	1.62	1.73	1.85	1.97	2.09	2.2	2.44	2.56	2.67	2.91	3.15	3.38	3.62	3.85	4.09	4.32
13	0.7	0.74	0.96	1.18	1.28	1.39	1.51	1.62	1.72	1.83	1.95	2.05	2.27	2.37	2.49	2.71	2.92	3.15	3.36	3.58	3.8	4.01
14	0.75	0.69	0.9	1.1	1.21	1.3	1.41	1.51	1.62	1.71	1.82	1.91	2.13	2.23	2.33	2.54	2.74	2.94	3.15	3.35	3.55	3.76
15	0.8	0.66	0.84	1.04	1.13	1.23	1.33	1.42	1.52	1.62	1.71	1.81	2	2.1	2.18	2.37	2.57	2.76	2.95	3.15	3.34	3.52
16	0.85	0.62	0.8	0.98	1.07	1.17	1.25	1.35	1.43	1.53	1.62	1.7	1.88	1.98	2.06	2.25	2.43	2.6	2.78	2.96	3.15	3.33
17	0.9	0.6	0.77	0.93	1.02	1.1	1.19	1.27	1.36	1.44	1.53	1.62	1.79	1.87	1.96	2.13	2.29	2.46	2.63	2.8	2.97	3.15
18	0.95	0.57	0.73	0.89	0.97	1.05	1.13	1.21	1.29	1.37	1.45	1.53	1.69	1.78	1.85	2.02	2.18	2.34	2.5	2.66	2.82	2.98
19	1	0.55	0.69	0.84	0.93	1.01	1.08	1.16	1.23	1.3	1.38	1.47	1.62	1.69	1.76	1.91	2.08	2.23	2.37	2.54	2.69	2.83

Cooper's 12-minute run field test

It is recommended that a lapped track or flat course be set out. The subject walks/runs as far as possible in 12 minutes and the distance covered is then recorded. Spiro *et al.*[13] showed a high correlation ($r = 0.897$) between distance covered in 12 minutes and $\dot{V}O_{2max}$. Table 8.6 provides predicted $\dot{V}O_{2max}$ scores from final distance achieved.

Table 8.6 Predicted $\dot{V}O_{2max}$ from distance covered in Cooper's 12-minute run field test. (From Cooper,[3] with permission)

Distance (miles)	Laps (1/4 mile track)	$\dot{V}O_{2max}$ (ml. kg^{-1}. min^{-1})
<1.0	<4	<25.0
1	4	25.0*
1.03		26.0*
1.07	4.25	27.0*
1.09		28.2
1.13	4.5	29
1.15		30.2
1.19	4.75	31.6
1.22		32.8
1.25	5	33.8
1.28		34.8
1.32	5.25	36.2
1.34		37
1.38	5.5	38.2
1.4		39.2
1.44	5.75	40.4
1.47		41.6
1.5	6	42.6
1.53		43.8
1.56	6.25	45
1.59		46
1.63	6.5	47.2
1.65		48
1.69	6.75	49.2
1.72		50.2
1.75	7	51.6
1.78		52.6
1.82	7.25	53.8
1.84		54.8
1.88	7.5	56
1.9		57
1.94	7.75	58.2
1.97		59.2
2	8	60.2

*Insufficient data at these distances to make reliable correlation's.

The McArdle step test

The McArdle step test is a 3-minute step test, originally designed using college gymnasium spectators' benches ($16\frac{1}{4}$ inches high) to allow for large numbers of subjects to be tested at once. Stepping is performed up and down on a single step in a four-step cycle, with the following cadences set by a metronome:

- men at 96 bpm or 24 steps per minute,
- women 88 bpm or 22 steps per minute.

At the end of the 3 minutes recovery heart rate is measured for 15 seconds from 5 to 20 seconds into recovery. This heart rate converted into beats per minute (bpm) is then entered into the following regression equations for predicting $\dot{V}O_{2max}$ for men and women, based on a 95% confidence that the scores will be within $\pm 16\%$ of actual $\dot{V}O_{2max}$. McArdle et al.[4] produced a table to circumvent use of the following equations, which predict $\dot{V}O_{2max}$ in $ml\,kg^{-1}\,min^{-1}$:

For men
$$\dot{V}O_{2max} = 111.33 - (0.42 \times \text{Step test heart rate, bpm})$$

For women
$$\dot{V}O_{2max} = 65.81 - (0.1847 \times \text{Step test heart rate, bpm})$$

The Chester step test

The Chester step test is a submaximal test, which makes it useful for untrained clients. It was developed at Chester College, UK, by Dr K. Sykes and is an incremental test, starting at a low pace with gradual increases and using either a 10-inch or a 12-inch step. It is at a present a part of the standard occupational health test for firefighters in the UK.

The Canadian standardized test of fitness step test

This test, originally developed for home use in 1967,[14,15] has received much attention for predicting $\dot{V}O_{2max}$ and providing prescribed exercise intensities.[5,16–20] It is an incremental test using two steps, starting at low intensities in relation to age and sex. At the end of each stage the subject's heart rate is measured and used to determine whether or not to continue to the next stage. The heart rate at the end of the final stage completed is entered into a calculation for predicting $\dot{V}O_{2max}$.

This test is available from: Fitness and Amateur Sport Canada, 365 Laurier Avenue West, Ottawa, Ontario, Canada K1A OX6.

The British NCF multi-stage fitness test

This test was originally developed by Leger and Lambert[6] at the University of Montreal, with the adaptations as described below by

Brewer *et al.*[7] at Loughborough University, UK. It consists of incremental stages of running back and forth between two markers 20 m apart, with the pace set by bleeps from a cassette tape. It is a maximal run which stops when the subject is no longer able to keep pace with the bleeps. $\dot{V}O_{2max}$ is predicted from a chart of the final stage and number of shuttles completed during that stage.

The test is available from: The National Coaching Foundation, 4 College Close, Beckett Park, Leeds, LS6 3QH, UK.

The Concept II rowing ergometer test for predicting $\dot{V}O_{2max}$

The protocol for this assessment developed by Lakomy and Lakomy[8] requires a 6-minute warm-up at 50–60% of predicted maximal heart rate (200 minus age). Following 2 minutes' recovery, the subject then rows for a 6-minute period at 80–90% of predicted maximum heart rate, keeping a constant 500 m split-time pace. By recording the distances covered and the heart rates attained during the test, the values are then used with a nomogram to predict $\dot{V}O_{2max}$.

Details of this test are available from: Concept II, 151–153, Nottingham Road, Old Basford, Nottingham, NG6 0FU, UK, or from the *Journal of Sports Sciences*, as referenced to Lakomy and Lakomy.[8]

Considerations for choosing the appropriate predictive $\dot{V}O_{2max}$ protocol

The Astrand submaximal cycle test, the Keele Lifestyle nomogram, the Chester step test and the Canadian step test allow the subject to start at a low intensity with successive increments and are thus very suitable for both sedentary and trained individuals of all ages.

The McArdle step test is beneficial for assessing large groups at the same time, but is not incremental, and therefore would be most suitable for either fit or young (e.g. school or college students) individuals.

Both the Cooper and Rockport tests provide for large group field assessments, but rely on individuals to select their own pace and require individuals to endure as fast a pace as possible. The elements of pacing experience and motivation may have an influence on end performance and thus predicted $\dot{V}O_{2max}$.

The NCF multi-stage fitness test is described as a progressive and maximal test, which also relies on motivation in the final stages but the pace is controlled. It seems well suited for young athletes, teams and more highly trained individuals.

The Cooper, Rockport and NCF tests all provide immediate feedback on performance in relation to other individuals, which can be useful for selection of potential athletes in competitive sport.

The Concept II rowing ergometer test is a sport-specific high-intensity test which is ideal for rowers and athletes, but may not be so suitable for general health-related assessments of older or sedentary individuals. The factor of training familiarity on this ergometer and muscular coordination will influence performance during this test.

The practicality of all the above protocols enables health and fitness professionals to possess a repertoire of tests which can be selected appropriate to age, sex, training status, and health and exercise goals, of clients, patients or athletes.

References

1. Astrand, P.O. and Ryhming, I. (1954) A nomogram for calculation of aerobic capacity from pulse rate during submaximal work. *J. Appl. Physiol.*, **7**, 218.
2. Kline, G.M., Porcari, J.P., Hintermeister, R. *et al.* (1987) Estimation of $\dot{V}O_{2max}$ from one-mile track walk, gender, age and body weight. *Med. Sci. Sports Exerc.*, **19**(3), 253–259.
3. Cooper, K.H. (1968) A means of assessing maximal oxygen uptake. *J. Am Med. Assoc.*, **203**, 201–204.
4. McArdle, W.D., Katch, F.I. and Katch, V.L. (1981) *Exercise Physiology – Energy Nutrition and Human Performance*, Lea and Febiger, New York.
5. Jette, M., Campbell, J., Mongeon, J. *et al.* (1976) The Canadian home fitness test as a predictor of aerobic capacity. *Can. Med. Assoc. J.*, **114**, 680–682.
6. Leger, L.A. and Lambert, J.A. (1982) A maximal multi-stage 20-m shuttle run test to predict $\dot{V}O_{2max}$. *Eur. J. Appl. Physiol.*, **49**, 1–12.
7. Brewer, J., Ramsbottom, R. and Williams, C. (1988) *A Progressive Shuttle Run Test for the Prediction of Maximum Oxygen Uptake*, The National Coaching Foundation Leeds, U.K. Copyright Loughborough University.
8. Lakomy, H.K.A. and Lakomy, J. (1993) Estimation of maximum oxygen uptake from submaximal exercise on a Concept II rowing ergometer. *J. Sports Sci.*, **11**, 227–232.
9. Sykes, K. (1995) The Chester Step Test. *J. Occ. Health*, Jan.
10. Astrand, P.O. and Rodahl, K. (1986) *Textbook of Work Physiology: Physiological Basis of Exercise*, 3rd edn, McGraw-Hill, London.
11. Buckley, J., Cannon, E. and Mapp, G. (1998) The development of a nomogram for predicting $\dot{V}O_{2max}$ from ratings of perceived exertion during submaximal exercise on a cycle ergometer *J. Sports Sci.*, **16**(i), 14–15.
12. Borg, G.A.V. (1982) Psychological basis of perceived exertion. *Med. Sci. Sports Exerc.*, **14**(5), 377–387.
13. Spiro, S.G., Juniper, E., Bowman, P. *et al.* (1974) Increasing work rate test for assessing the physiological strain of submaximal exercise. *Clin. Sci Molec. Med.*, **46**, 191–206.
14. Bailey, D.A., Shephard, R.J. and Mirwald, R.L. (1967) Validation of a self administered home test of cardiorespiratory fitness. *Can. J. Appl. Sports Sci.*, **1**, 67.
15. Shepard, R.J., Bailey, R.A. and Mirwald, R.L. (1976) Development of the Canadian home fitness test. *Can. Med. Assoc. J.*, **114**, 680.
16. Jette, M. (1977) A calculator to predict maximal oxygen uptake for use in conjunction with the Canadian home fitness test. *Can. J. Pub. Hlth*, **68**, 195–198.
17. Bonen, A., Gardner, J., Primrose, J. *et al.* (1977) An evaluation of the Canadian home fitness test. *Can. J. Appl. Sports Sci.*, **21**, 133–136.

18. Jette, M. (1978) The standardised test of fitness in occupational health: a pilot project. *Can. J. Public Hlth*, **69**, 431–438.
19. Jette, M. (1979) Comparison between predicted $\dot{V}O_{2max}$ from the Astrand procedure and the Canadian home fitness test. *Can. J. Appl. Sports Sci.*, **4**(3), 214–218.
20. Jette, M. (1983) The energy requirements of the Canadian home fitness test and their application to the evaluation of work performance. *Can. J. Public Hlth*, **74**, 401–403.

9

User friendly tables and charts for prescribing exercise with aerobic equipment

The physiological basis of exercise prescription intensities (pace) in relation to $\dot{V}O_{2max}$ and training status
User friendly charts for prescribing exercise intensities
Chapter summary
References

The physiological basis of exercise prescription intensities (pace) in relation to $\dot{V}O_{2max}$ and training status

Sustainable beneficial aerobic exercise for improving cardiorespiratory fitness occurs at 55–65%, 65–75% and 75–90% of $\dot{V}O_{2max}$ for sedentary, moderately active and highly active trained individuals, respectively.[1,2] In Chapter 7 it was noted that setting the right intensity, especially with a sedentary individual, is probably the hardest part of establishing an exercise prescription. For the newcomer, if the initial pace or intensity is slightly too high, this may cause them not to maintain the exercise long enough, thus imparting a sense of failure. If the pace is too slow with some individuals, they may possibly feel a lack of achievement.

Pace and oxygen uptake

Walking/running pace

The relationship between pace and oxygen uptake has been shown to be that for every 1 kph of walking or running pace, 3–3.5 ml kg^{-1} min^{-1} of

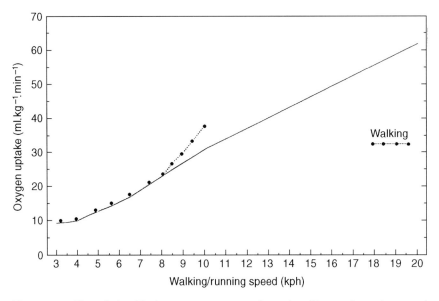

Figure 9.1 The relationship between oxygen uptake and walking and running speed. (Adapted from Falls and Humphrey,[4] Menier and Pugh[5] and Margaria et al.[6])

oxygen uptake is required.[1,3–6] These factors are, however, assumed for adults walking/running on the flat at speeds >3.5 kph, where the exercise is submaximal and with minimal head wind resistance. The motorized treadmill is ideally suited for fulfilling these assumptions. Furthermore, in order for a reasonable linear relationship to be maintained between pace and oxygen uptake, there must be a transition from walking to running at 7.5–8.0 kph.[1,3–6] If walking were attempted above this speed, then oxygen uptake would increase in a pronounced curvilinear manner with any further increase in walking speed (Figure 9.1). When running at higher velocities (>12 kph), stride length has also been shown to noticeably influence efficiency of oxygen uptake.[7] Table 9.1 provides subjective descriptions of walking/jogging/running in relation to speed (kph and minutes per mile). Figure 9.1 and Table 9.2 are based on the relationship between pace and oxygen consumption.

Exercise cycle ergometer workrate

For exercise cycle ergometers, an oxygen consumption of about 1 litre min^{-1} is required for every 70 W of pedalling workrate.[1] During seated exercise on a cycle ergometer, body weight does not greatly affect workrate, except in obese individuals, and therefore oxygen consumption can usually be described in absolute terms (litres min^{-1}). Figure 9.2 and Table 9.3 are based on the relationship between cycle ergometer workrate and oxygen consumption.

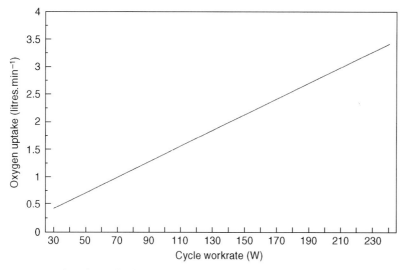

Figure 9.2 The relationship between oxygen uptake and workrate on the cycle ergometer. (Adapted from Astrand and Rodahl.[7])

Rowing ergometer pace

Unlike treadmill running or exercise cycling, Lakomy and Lakomy[8] described ergometer rowing (the Concept II model) as having a curvilinear increasing oxygen cost with any given increase in workrate pace. Furthermore, this study showed that non-rowers required more oxygen per given workrate pace than experienced oarsmen. Two different mathematical equations describing oxygen usage for rowers and non-rowers have been derived, [8] as illustrated in Figure 9.3, which have been used to determine the prescription values in Table 9.4 and 9.5:

For non-rowers: $\dot{V}O_2 = 0.114 \times speed^{2.42}$
For experienced oarsmen $\dot{V}O_2 = 0.102 \times speed^{2.42}$

Speed measured in metres per second.

User friendly charts for prescribing exercise intensity

The following charts and tables can be used where $\dot{V}O_{2max}$ has either been measured or predicted. The prescriptions for exercise cycle ergometers may be more representative when $\dot{V}O_{2max}$ is attained from a cycle test and the prescriptions for walking/jogging/running may be more representative from treadmill, step tests and walking/running field tests.

Tables 9.2–9.5 provide paces, speeds and workrates for treadmill walking/running, cycle ergometers and rowing ergometers. An appropriate exercise intensity (pace or workrate) prescription for these activities is established by:

- determining the individual's $\dot{V}O_{2max}$ (see Chapter 8),
- locating their $\dot{V}O_{2max}$ on the chart,

- from their $\dot{V}O_{2max}$ score reading across to the training status column, which best describes the individual subject/client.

Exercise prescription for improving cardiorespiratory fitness

Exercising at the paces determined from the user friendly charts should be performed for 15 or more minutes, continuously, at least 2–3 times per week to create a training effect.[2,9] Within a gymnasium setting, the 15 + minutes can be divided among treadmills, cycles and rowing ergometers, to engage a variety of large muscle groups and prevent the boredom of having to sustain a single activity. If one of the objectives is to change body composition through decreased adipose fat, then increased frequency, duration and possibly lowered intensity of participation will be required. When adherence to regular exercise occurs, then retests and follow-up prescriptions must consider both changes in $\dot{V}O_{2max}$ and training status (i.e. from

Table 9.1 Descriptions of walk/run pacing

Subjective pace rating for healthy person	Actual pace	
	(kph)	(mins/mile)
Good strolling walk	3.0–5.0	25:00–19:24
Brisk walk	5.5–7.0	17:36–13:38
Slow jog	7.5–8.0	12:54–12:06
Moderate jog/slow run	8.5–10	11:23–9:41
Running	10.5 +	9:13 +

Table 9.2 Prescribed walking/jogging/running paces in relation to $\dot{V}O_{2max}$ and training status

	Training status		
	Sedentary	Moderate/regularly active	Highly/well trained
$\dot{V}O_{2max}$ (ml kg^{-1} min^{-1})	Pace at 55–65% $\dot{V}O_{2max}$ (kph) (min/mile)	Pace at 65–75% $\dot{V}O_{2max}$ (kph) (min/mile)	Pace at 75–90% $\dot{V}O_{2max}$ (kph) (min/mile)
20–25	4.2 (23:00)	5.0 (19:24)	–
26–30	5.5 (17:36)	6.5 (14:54)	–
31–35	6.5 (14:43)	7.7 (12:34)	–
36–40	7.5 (12:54)	9.0 (10:45)	9.7 (9:58)
41–45	8.6 (11:15)	10.2 (9:29)	11.1 (8:43)
46–50	9.6 (10:05)	11.5 (8:25)	12.4 (7:48)
51–55	10.7 (9:02)	12.3 (7:37)	13.7 (7:04)
56–60	11.7 (8:16)	14.0 (6:55)	15.0 (6:27)
61–65	12.8 (7:34)	15.2 (6:22)	16.5 (5:52)
66 +	13.8 (7:01)	16.5 (5:52)	17.8 (5:26)

Table 9.3   Prescribed exercise cycle ergometer work rates in relation to $\dot{V}O_{2max}$ and training status

Workrate at $\dot{V}O_{2max}$ (litres. min^{-1})	Training status		
	Sedentary	Moderate/regularly active	Highly/well trained
	Workrate at 55–65% $\dot{V}O_{2max}$ (Watts)	Workrate at 65–75% $\dot{V}O_{2max}$ (Watts)	75–85% $\dot{V}O_{2max}$ (Watts)
0.9–1.1	36	41	–
1.2–1.4	43	50	–
1.5–1.7	65	75	–
1.8–2.0	84	96	102
2.1–2.3	97	112	119
2.4–2.7	111	127	136
2.8–3.0	129	149	159
3.1–3.3	143	165	176
3.4–3.6	157	181	192
3.7–3.9	171	196	210
4.0–4.2	185	213	227
4.3–4.5	195	226	240
4.6–4.8	209	241	257
4.9–5.1	223	257	274
5.2 +	236	273	291

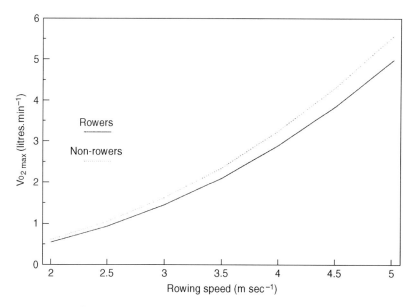

Figure 9.3   The oxygen cost of ergometer rowing – Concept II model. (Adapted from Lakomy and Lakomy.[8])

Table 9.4 Prescribed rowing ergometer paces (Concept II model) in relation to $\dot{V}O_{2max}$ and training status (for experienced Oarsmen). (Adapted from Lakomy and Lakomy[8])

$\dot{V}O_{2max}$ (litres min^{-1})	Rowing pace 500 m split-time (min:sec) For less trained 65–75% $\dot{V}O_{2max}$	Rowing pace 500 m split-time (min:sec) For well trained 75–85% $\dot{V}O_{2max}$
2.0–2.2	2:50–2:45	2:40–2:35
2.3–2.5	2:40–2:35	2:35–2:30
2.6–2.8	2:20–2:25	2:25–2:20
2.9–3.1	2:25–2:20	2:20–2:15
3.2–3.4	2:20–2:15	2:15–2:10
3.5–3.7	2:15–2:10	2:10–2:05
3.8–4.0	2:10–2:05	2:05–2:00
4.1–4.3	2:05–2:00	2:00–1:55
4.4–4.6	2:00–1:55	1:55–1:50
4.7–4.9	1:55–1:53	1:52
5.0–5.2	1:53	1:50
5.3–5.5	1:52	1:48
5.6–5.8	1:50	1:45
5.9–6.1	1:43	1:40
6.2 +	1:40	1:35

Table 9.5 Prescribed rowing ergometer paces (Concept II model) in relation to $\dot{V}O_{2max}$ and training status (for non-rowers). (Adapted from Lakomy and Lakomy[8])

$\dot{V}O_{2max}$ (litres min^{-1})	Rowing pace 500 m split-time (min:sec) For sedentary 55–65% $\dot{V}O_{2max}$	Rowing pace 500 m split-time (min:sec) For moderately trained 65–75% $\dot{V}O_{2max}$	Rowing pace 500 m split-time (min:sec) For well trained 75–85% $\dot{V}O_{2max}$
1.1–1.3	4:00–3:55	3:40–3:35	3:25–3:20
1.4–1.6	3:35–3:30	3:25–3:20	2:10–3:05
1.7–1.9	320–315	3:10–3:05	3:00–2:55
2.0–2.2	3:10–3:05	3:00–2:55	2:50–2:45
2.3–2.5	3:00–2:55	2:50–2:45	2:40–2:35
2.6–2.8	2:50–2:45	2:35–2:30	2:30–2:25
2.9–3.1	2:40–2:35	2:30–2:25	2:25–2:20
3.2–3.4	2:35–2:30	2:25–2:20	2:20–2:15
3.5–3.7	2:25–2:20	2:20–2:15	2:15–2:10
3.8–4.0	2:20–2:15	2:15–2:10	2:10–2:05
4.1–4.3	2:15	2:10	2:05
4.4–4.6	2:10	2:05	2:00
4.7–4.9	2:05	2:03	1:58
5.0–5.2	2:00	1:58	1:54
5.3–5.5	1:58	1:56	1:52
5.6 +	1:56	1:53	1:50

sedentary to moderately active). As thoroughly discussed in Chapter 3, long-term adherence, however, relies not just on objective feedback of increased fitness performance but also on an awareness of a variety of psychosocial factors, including: self-efficacy, previous experience with exercise, knowledge of health-exercise benefits, group versus individual activities, and age and susceptibility to illness.[10–12]

Chapter summary

A variety of maximal and submaximal protocols for predicting $\dot{V}O_{2max}$, outlined in this Chapter, provide exercise health professionals with the opportunity to select tests appropriate to age, sex, training status and fitness objectives. For purposes of health-related fitness, as discussed in Chapters 1–3, 7 and 12, the assessment is aimed to assist in client compliance through providing suitable and achievable intensities of exercise alongside considerations of frequency and duration of an agreeable activity mode(s). The user friendly charts in this chapter have thus been developed to allow a variety of health professionals (fitness consultants, doctors, nurses, physiotherapists, community health promoters) to more easily prescribe beneficial aerobic exercise on cycle ergometers, rowers and treadmills when a $\dot{V}O_{2max}$ score has either been measured or predicted.

References

1. Astrand, P.O. and Rodahl, K. (1986) *Textbook of Work Physiology: Physiological Basis of Exercise*, 3rd edn, McGraw-Hill, New York.
2. American College of Sports Medicine (1990) Position Stand: The recommended quantity and quality of exercise for developing and maintaining cardiorespiratory and muscular fitness in healthy adults. *Med. Sci. Sports Exerc.*, **22**(2), 265–274.
3. Williams, C. (1985) Nutritional aspects of exercise induced fatigue. *Proc. Nutrition Soc.*, **44**, 245–256.
4. Falls, H.B. and Humphrey L.D. (1976). Energy cost of running and walking in young women. *Med. Sci. Sports Exerc.*, **8**, 9–14.
5. Menier, D.R. and Pugh, L.G.C.E. (1968) The relation of oxygen intake and velocity of walking and running in competition walkers. *J. Physiol.*, **197**, 717–721.
6. Margaria, R., Cerritelli, P., Aghemo, P. *et al.* (1963) Energy cost of running. *J. Appl. Physiol.*, **18**, 367–370.
7. Hogberg, P. (1952) How do the stride length and stride frequency influence the energy output during running? *Arbeitphysiol.*, **14**, 431.
8. Lakomy, H.K.A. and Lakomy, J. (1993) Estimation of maximum oxygen uptake from submaximal exercise on a Concept II rowing ergometer. *J. Sports Sci.*, **11**, 227–232.
9. McArdle, W.D., Katch, F.L. and Katch, V.L. (1981) *Exercise Physiology – Energy Nutrition and Human Performance*, Lea and Febiger, New York.
10. Boyd, L. and Nielsen, C.C. (1979) Factors affecting health club attendance: a comparison of simple and elaborate settings. *J. Sports Med. Phys. Fit.*, **29**(4), 310–313.

11. Kariska, A.M., Bayles, C., Cauley, J. *et al.* (1986) A randomised exercise trial in older women: increased activity over two years and the factors associated with compliance. *Med. Sci. Sports Exerc.*, **18**(5), 557–562.

12. Sallis, J.F., Haskill, W.L., Fortmann, S.P. *et al.* (1986) Predictors of adoption and maintenance of physical activity in a community sample. *Prevent. Med.*, **15**, 331–341.

10

Muscle, bone and joint considerations for cardiovascular exercise

Responses and adaptations of the muscles, bones and joints
Preventing muscle, bone and joint problems in the newcomer
Acknowledging weight-bearing and non-weight-bearing activities
Posture and the spine–lower limb interface during various aerobic activities

This chapter serves to acknowledge the fact that if an individual is going to become more active, then whatever mode of activity they choose, the movements required will always be limited by their ability to sustain the coordinated actions of the muscles, bones and joints. It is not a chapter designed to act as a guide to teaching the correct technique of numerous forms of activities for cardiovascular health, for this is left to specialist training courses and teaching manuals. A number of typical aerobic activities, however, will be used as examples to highlight some common problems, misconceptions and useful guidance tips. These will include cycling (static or bicycle), exercising on stepper machines, walking/jogging/running (on the road or a treadmill), swimming, using rowing machines, and dance-type aerobic and step aerobic exercising to music.

When movements are performed properly and effectively, taking into account any pre-existing physical condition, the amount of benefit and enjoyment can be optimized. There are a number of factors which can either *enhance*, *diminish* or *interfere* with the ability to perform movement effectively, as illustrated in Figure 10.1, and which are acquired for various reasons, including:

- naturally (via genetics, age and gender),
- through practice/participation or non-participation,
- as a result of poor practice/technique,
- from a disease, accident or ailment,
- simply from the process of ageing.

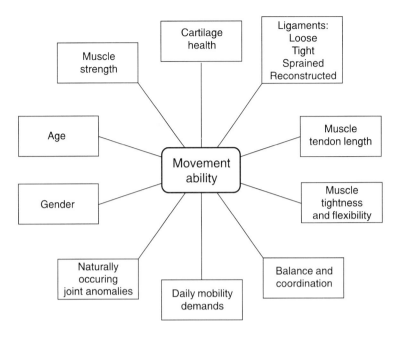

Figure 10.1 Factors which affect movement ability.

Whether naturally occurring or owing to one's actions of daily living the above factors are related to:

- muscle strength,
- available joint range of movement,
- ligament and tendon integrity (tight, loose, injured, sprained or strained),
- joint cartilage integrity and osteoarthritis of the hips or knees,
- the inability to bear weight fully on the lower limbs for any reason.

In many cases the chosen mode of activity(ies) has to acknowledge that the client's balance and coordination may also be hampered by the above factors.

Responses and adaptations of the muscles, bones and joints (the musculoskeletal system)

The system of muscles, bones and joints (the musculoskeletal system), like the cardiovascular system, responds and adapts to physical activity. What must be appreciated is that bones and joints are possibly more vulnerable to being overstressed and becoming injured as compared to the cardiovascular system. It is easier to protect against overstressing the cardiovascular system because heart rate and breathing rate provide a constant 'inbuilt' feedback and monitoring mechanism. The only practical gauge for monitoring the amount of stress being applied to the musculoskeletal system during activity is the presence of a pain or an ache. The presence of pain either means an injury has occurred or that some disorder is present that could potentially lead to a problem.

This lack of any practical monitoring system means that even before any pain begins to arise the process of trauma or degeneration of a bone or joint tissue can already be in progress. Often pains associated with 'over-use' musculoskeletal injuries (e.g. knee cap problems or shin splints from brisk walking or jogging, and shoulder problems from swimming) possibly do not appear until it is too late and then that form of activity has to either be altered, decreased or stopped completely. One problem of dealing with a person with an injury, which requires them to alter their amount or mode of exercise, is that it presents the exercise professional with not just having to deal with the physical injury but the corresponding psychological hurdle in getting the client to accept altering or temporarily stopping something they enjoy. When this problem occurs in a person fairly new to a regular exercise programme, but where they have not yet reached the maintenance stage in their exercise behaviour, the perceived feeling of well-being and confidence can easily be 'knocked' and they are likely to relapse to a stage of having to recontemplate their exercise participation (see stages of change model, Chapter 3, Figure 3.4). The next section of this chapter will address how such a situation can arise and how possibly to prevent it.

Preventing muscle, bone and joint problems in the newcomer

Much of this book is aimed at guiding the previously sedentary individual onto the 'right path' towards a healthier more active life. Joint problems or disease, injury, pain, previous surgery or osteoporosis, coupled with a lack of confidence and coordination in the potential newcomer client (contemplation to action stage), may be perceived as a barrier to participate in activity, as noted in Chapter 3. As discussed in Chapter 12, during the consultation process any musculoskeletal limitations will be acknowledged and the activities chosen will respect these limitations and hopefully the related perceived barriers to activity will be removed. From the perspective of the exercise professional, the problem may lie not in the injured or *less well* joints, but in the concern over those muscles and joints which are apparently healthy. The following example describes why exercise professionals must acknowledge the potential problem in the healthy but 'unfit' muscles and joints.

When a sedentary person takes up regular activity or exercise to a level which can improve aerobic fitness, it is quite possible that this improvement (an increase in VO_{2max} by $10-25\%$) can occur within as short a period as 8 weeks (see Chapter 4). The sense of well-being that often corresponds to such an achievement can provide a level of both the confidence and fitness for an individual to want to exercise longer, harder and more frequently. Such a progression is obviously beneficial to both the short-term and potential longer term health of the cardiovascular system (heart, blood vessels, circulation, and blood), but can the same be said for the bones and joints? Here is a clear example of where the progression of an individual's programme is not limited by their cardio-vascular or psychological fitness, but by the fact that the bones, tendons, ligaments and cartilage which make up a joint need longer to adapt to increased participation than the cardiovascular system. This must clearly be explained to the client in order to avoid the future disappointment of their having to alter or reduce their programme from what could have been a preventable over-use injury. Injury-forced relapse in exercise behaviour could cause a great sense of 'undoing' some of the cardiovascular and psychological benefits for which they have worked so hard to achieve.

Acknowledging weight-bearing and non-weight-bearing modes of activity

The effects of gravity greatly influence the ability of muscles and joints of the lower limb to perform activity. In the heavier person, body weight significantly adds much more resistance to performance as compared with a lighter person. It must be remembered that a person who is heavy due to excess fat probably does not have any larger or stronger bones and joints than a lighter individual; the bone and joint integrity may not be in proportion to the heavier individual's weight. Activities like exercise cycling and using rowing machines unload the joints to a great degree because the foot and the pelvis are supported simultaneously by the cycle pedal and seat, respectively. The resistance set using these machines is much less dependent on body weight and allows the intensity of activity to be set much more easily and controllable relative to cardiovascular fitness, but with much of the joint stress removed. It takes longer for joints to adapt to increased activity than it does for the cardiocvascular system and muscles.

Neck and back problems

A commonly encountered perceived barrier to exercise participation and often a sequel to poor exercise technique is neck and low back pain. With a careful choice of activity, exacerbation of the problems can be avoided. Furthermore, poor technique when performing an activity is in itself a cause of back and neck problems. Sometimes a client will complain of increasing aches and pains during or following their exercise session, but was this due to the exercise or some other prior event (e.g. a long drive in the car, home decorating or gardening activities, lifting of awkward heavy objects)? It is important to ask exactly what the client has been doing other than their exercise. It must also be remembered that warmth is a pain reliever in itself. During exercise the body becomes much warmer and it is not until hours later, once the body has cooled, that pain appears to signal that a problem is present; the problem may have been present during exercise but the pain was masked by body warmth.

If at all possible, collaborating with or having available advice from a physiotherapist is highly advantageous. The term *neck and back problems* is very wide-ranging and just because two people have the same ache or pain arising from the same spot does not necessarily mean that they will have the same problem. Essentially, pains in the spine can arise from muscle, bone, vertebrae or discs, nerve dysfunction, ligament strain, or an impact or whiplash displacement of vertebrae. In some cases a particular movement or activity will benefit or at least not exacerbate a problem, whereas in other cases it will be strictly forbidden. With some conditions there may be the possibility to take up a particular activity in the future once the problem is resolved, but in other cases a particular activity or exercise will never be an option. Be prepared and get some collaborative advice from a physiotherapist who understands sports and exercise movements, because these are the types of problems or questions a client will want clearly answered.

Posture and the spine – lower limb interface during various aerobic activities

The word 'posture' is a very common term and the average person will associate it with sitting up straight, with the chest pushed slightly forward, the stomach held in and the chin slightly tucked. Such recommendations may be fine while one is sitting still, but during any activity and especially aerobic-type exercise such rigidity may restrict the effective expansion and contraction of the rib cage and the rise and fall of the diaphagm in order to achieve unrestricted breathing. General recommendations on posture during dynamic exercise should include:

- avoiding any excessive backward extension or forward flexion of the spine,
- avoiding forward and backward movement of the neck, where the chin is frequently poked forward and then retracted.

The recommendations above are most important when the hips, knees and ankles are sequentially being flexed and extended for a given duration. The stable foundation which allows lower limb human movement to occur is the combined semi-rigid structures of the spine/pelvis and the rigid elements of the ground or pedal to which the foot is in contact. Without a stable spine, pelvis and low back, muscle action will be inefficient and less effective. Muscle tension is not the only form of stress being applied to the spine during sequential lower limb activity – there is also the stress and strains on the nerve fibres which run down inside the spine and down the length of the legs that control these muscles. Extra movements of the head and neck or excessive unnecessary flexion or extension of the lower spine will further contribute to stress on the nerve fibres. Typical examples of poor musculoskeletal movements are highlighted in the following activities, with points and recommendations found in Table 10.1.

In the following examples of activities, it is assumed that the points discussed will be implemented in light of the fact that the instructor, coach or supervisor in each of these activities is suitably trained and experienced.

Table 10.1   Movement considerations during various cardiovascular/aerobic activities

Activity/exercise	Amount of impact	Degree of weight-bearing	Range of movement (ROM) required
Treadmill	Increases with pace/speed	Full	Relatively little required in the lower limb, apart from the ankle which needs good dorsiflexion for the swing-through phase of walking
Stepper	Minimal	Usually full weight-bearing, but arms can be used to take some of the load Can be reduced or removed if seat/perch is available	Can be adjusted
Rower	None	Minimal (a seated activity)	Can be used with relatively little ROM in lower limbs The upper limbs need grip strength and shoulder movement to the horizontal Elbow ROM will affect the stroke
Static bicycle	None	Minimal	> 90 degrees knee flexion required
Swimming	None	None	Good shoulder and hip movement required, but flotation devices can be used for assistance or to immobilize an injured joint
Aerobics	Low to high	Full	Adapted moves can be used
Step aerobics	Designed to be low impact but very high impacts often occur	Full	Pain-free knee flexion and ankle movements sufficient to use a step; step height can be altered to accommodate some restriction of ankle, knees and hip

Walking and running

During walking or running, leaning forward too much is often found on a treadmill, where a person leans on the handrails, their bottom is pushed out, and thus an extra amount of tension is present down the whole length of the spine and right down the back of the legs. During treadmill exercise, arm swing should be encouraged as soon as the client is happy to let go of the handrails, as this will allow normal reciprocal movements of the upper limbs and shoulders in response, to balance the forces created by the lower limbs naturally.

The persistence of any gait pattern abnormalities (e.g. limping) will place abnormal stresses on the lower limbs, which may transmit stress higher up the body to the back and neck and compensatory movements may occur which in themself create extra stress.

The added impact of running, that may be desirable with improved fitness, may exacerbate neck or back problems. Treadmills with a mechanism to create an uphill gradient can be set so that the client is walking but the intensity is similar to their running on the flat.

As neck and back problems are very common, the continuation of aerobic exercises by the use of less- or non-impact activity modes is an obvious option. For those who would describe themselves as 'a runner' or involved in a sport relying on running and who wish to keep fit during a period of neck or back trouble, then some of the activities described next may be suitable alternatives.

Rowing

On a rowing machine, common faults are:

- Leaning back too much to create extra propulsion.
- Poking, the head and neck forward, which combined with the arm action can stress the upper spine (between the shoulder-blades).

Also during rowing, the hips and knees are greatly flexed on the initial 'catch phase', and if at the same time the spine is hunched forward too much again the combined position of the flexed hips and the hunched spine creates extra tension in the nerve fibres down the spine and through the pelvis.

Rowing is a low-impact, non-weight-bearing activity and can be useful where pain, joint tissue integrity and reduced joint range of movement limits one's abilities in other activities.

In the case of an injury where one leg is immobile, the activity can still be performed where there has been injury/surgery to the knee or ankle. Rowing can still be performed with the non-injured leg and the arms while the injured leg is immobilized, as seen in Figure 10.2. Aerobic fitness and cardiovascular health can still be maintained during the rehabilitation of the injured body segment and then the injured limb can be introduced progressively into the rowing activity as required.

Following, or in the presence of, upper limb problems, use of a rowing machine needs to be carefully assessed. After a suitable period of time following fractures (breaks) or surgery, care must be taken but does not always preclude its use. Collaborative medical advice should always be sought in order to determine the suitability of participating in this activity. The same precautions should be taken if neck or back problems, such as sciatica, are present.

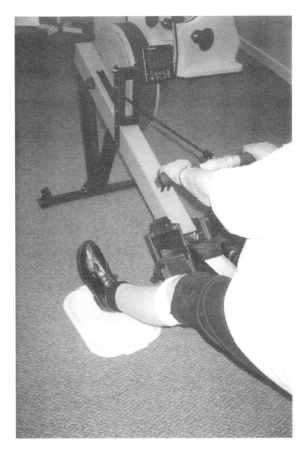

Figure 10.2 One legged rowing due to knee and ankle immobilized from an injury or prosthetic limb. With the foot on a plastic tray, there is low friction between the foot and floor which allows the leg to slide back and forth easily. A beneficial aerobic exercise session is performed.

Step-ups

On a stepping machine the initial skill of learning this activity often forces an individual to lean forward onto their arms and push their buttocks outwards, causing tension down the spine and down the back of the legs. Further compounding problems with the stepper is the fact that the client may, for some reason, forget to relieve the muscle tension in the lifting leg while the opposing leg is pushing downwards on the pedal. With little relief of tension in both the leg's, quadriceps and the hamstrings, the hip and knee joints are tightened and acute pain in the knee cap and low back can often prevail. Success or failure with the stepping machine is a matter of skill and coordination. In the early stages, however, when individuals struggle a little with this skill, they quickly perceive the onset of heavier breathing as a result of lack of fitness and yet when they pedalled an exercise cycle at the same relative intensity they were in much more control of the action and their breathing rate was controllable. Spending time carefully to instruct a client on this piece of equipment will prevent overstressing both the musculoskeletal and cardiovascular systems, which will result in the client succeeding and benefiting.

Common faults when using the stepper and the appropriate corrections are as follows:

Fault. Unequal stepping, where one lower limb moves through a greater range of movement than the other, and unequal pressure is exerted by the limbs; often compensatory movements of the upper body will be seen at the same time.
Correction. The stepping height should be reduced so that movement is symmetrical.

Fault. Rising onto the toes, failing to keep the whole foot on the step, can lead to calf muscle or Achilles' tendon strain.
Correction. Encourage the distribution of weight over the arch of the foot, and keeping the heel down.

Fault. Too much hip flexion and/or sticking the bottom out. Apart from the lower back strain involved, often the neck is placed in a position where the chin is poking forward and the head tilts backwards in order for the client to look up in front of them. This posture often coincides with holding onto the stepper handrails which can lead to raised shoulders and tense upper limb muscles. This will further aggravate any neck problems.
Correction. Tuck in the abdomen and bottom when stepping, and keep the head level and shoulders relaxed with a light grip on the handrails.

Using a stepper causes much less impact than running, although the actions are very similar. It is a 'kinetic chain' and a 'functional' exercise, which means it involves the coordinated and simultaneous actions of a number of joints and muscles resembling normal daily movement requirements.

Some steppers have a seat/perch, where the client sits down the opposite way to if they were standing on the pedals (Figure 10.3). The pumping leg action is very similar, but the seat can provide partial or full weight-bearing activity, like an exercise cycle, and it is easier to limit range of movement to avoid pain, or accommodate for an injury or weakness of the lower limb. As strength and range of movement are improved and pain decreased, the client may be able to progress towards standing and performing the more normal stepping activity. The seat/perch can enable a functional aerobic exercise to be maintained throughout rehabilitation, in the presence of existing orthopaedic problems, or could even be used by stroke or head injury patients who have enough leg strength to move the pedals but have no coordination, or balance preventing them from being able to stand up.

The seat/perch also allows for lower limb exercise using large muscle groups, although their normal daily function is compromised.

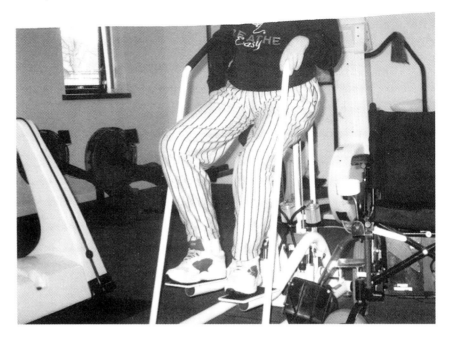

Figure 10.3 This client has suffered a head injury and although has some strength and movement in the legs, all function of balance and coordination has been lost and she is unable to stand. The seat perch allows the large muscles of the legs to be exercised which not only has cardiovascular exercise benefits but also the psycho-social benefits of participating in a typical and positive health environment.

Nevertheless, the exercise can have benefits to cardiovascular health as well as the psychosocial benefits the client gains from participation.

Exercise cycling

On an bicycle or exercise cycle, similar principles apply to the position-ing and movement of the back and neck as in the use of the rowing machine and stepper. The same tension in the spine, pelvis and down the back of the legs can prevail from the hunching over of firmly grasped handlebars in the the non-cyclist (those who are not highly trained at the sport of cycle racing).

Ensuring the correct saddle height can prevent excessive stress on the knee cap and in the Achilles' tendon/calf muscle area. The saddle should be adjusted so that when the the pedal is at its lowest point, the knee should be slightly bent. If the handlebars are too far forward, resulting in a 'stretched' riding position, the neck may be extended forward and tilted backwards and the lower back excessively flexed, with the associated problems as stated earlier. It is not uncommon for these two faults to arise. Exercisers often do not bother to adjust the cycle to suit themselves after a previous user, or they may not be made aware that the riding position can be altered, or they simply cannot be bothered to ask for help with the adjustments. Even worse is the non-supervised situation, where no one is sufficiently knowledgeable or available to assist.

Pedal speed for non-cyclists is typically between 50 and 75 pedals per minute or revolutions per minute (rpm). If the resistance is too high, it will manifest in the inability to work within this pedal speed, and an asymmetrical action may use less effective muscles of the legs and the pelvis. It is important to aim to perform cycling with equal pressure from both limbs; if this cannot be achieved, there is the need for an adjustment of cycling position or pace to allow the weaker side to match the stronger side. This is often seen when clients have low back pain, sciatica or arthritis of the hip; compensatory upper body movements give a clear sign that this is occurring.

The cycle, like the stepping machine, is a non-impact, 'kinetic chain' type of exercise, but its use depends upon the ability to flex the knee joint to at least 90 degrees. Upper limb problems should not preclude the use of a static bicycle. The handlebars can be adjusted to lie nearer to the rider, so that if there is an upper limb problem the rider can rest the affected arm upon the handlebar if needed.

Swimming

Swimming is considered to be a non-impact, low joint stress exercise. Individuals often choose to perform the most traditional of all strokes, the breast stroke, because of the following advantages over other strokes: easier flotation, easier breathing, the intermittent action of a stroking and gliding phase, and possibly preventing getting the hair wet. One problem is that it may result in swimming with the head out of the water, causing the neck to be acutely extended backwards and the low back to be arched (hyperextended). Potentially this positioning can lead to further problems for those with existing neck or back trouble.

Swimming may still be an option even if shoulder or arm movement is restricted, for example in an individual with arthritis or a stroke. Extra flotation may be used to compensate for reduced arm action, or other adaptations may be needed to suit the client

Coaching should ensure the correct technique during breast stroke, with the head lower in the water during the glide phase of the arm stroke and using a variety of different strokes to engage different muscle actions. The crawl stroke, generally requires the face to be in the water and automatically changes the neck and back position into a less hyperextended position.

Swimming is often chosen because the pressure on the joints is relieved as compared to land-based activities. If performed correctly, the level of intensity can be controlled from very low-energy to very high-energy expenditures, but incorrect posture and technique are just as likely to cause pain and injury as land-based activities.

Even if an individual has upper limb problems, swimming still provides good exercise if the arms and upper body are supported by a flotation device and the legs are left to perform the activity. This rationale can be reversed if lower limb problems exist, where a flotation device can support the lower limbs and the upper limbs perform the exercise.

Aerobics – exercise/dance to music

Aerobics is a full weight-bearing activity, and can be performed using low- to high-impact movements and at a wide range of intensities. An effective instructor should be able to guide and individualize the intensity for each participant in a class, in spite of the music tempo being the same for everyone. In a class-based activity, it is the speed and range of limb actions which dictate the intensity. Smaller range movements are associated with low-impact exercise. It must be appreciated that the less experienced participant will be more likely to follow the instructor while the more advanced participant may perform the action to the level of impact or intensity which is most suitable to them. Properly trained instructors are able to adapt or provide alternative moves or sequences to cater for individuals with particular problems such as pain, weakness or reduced range of movement.

Some of the key instructing points when considering individuals with potential or existing musculoskeletal problems include:

- preventing the 'locking-out' of joints – taking joints (particularly the knee and elbow) rapidly to the end of their range of movement without control,
- poking out the chin – the neck should not be forward of the shoulders,
- rounding or hunching the shoulders,
- 'sticking out' the bottom – corrected by a balance between abdominal and gluteal muscles,
- continual unnecessary bouncing on the toes, leading to Achilles' tendon and calf muscle strain, can occur even after just one class,
- bouncing into stretches, rather than easing into them slowly and with control,
- attempting to stretch a muscle too far, which may overstrain the muscle tendon, ligaments and joint capsule tissues.

During most exercises in an aerobics class, except in specific actions where trunk and/or hip flexion are required, the trunk should be in an erect position, with the bottom tucked in. This does not imply that a rigid posture should be adopted, but merely that a good posture should be returned to and maintained where possible.

Step aerobics

Step aerobics was originally conceived as a low-impact activity, where the intensity could be increased by raising the height of the step as opposed to increasing the speed and impact of the movement. It has now evolved to include elaborate choreography which requires propelling oneself into the air, around and off the step. Thus more advanced classes actually involve a higher impact than can be achieved in any non-step based aerobics session.

The same demonstration and teaching techniques apply as in aerobics, but with some added concerns:

- not putting the whole foot onto the platform – repetition of this can result in foot strain,
- not putting the heel down in the land phase – this can result in the Achilles' tendon and/or calf muscle never being put into a relaxed state and thus being under constant strain or tension,
- looking at the feet, floor and step in the learning stages – this leads to the head dropping and incorrect posture of the whole spine and lower back.

Footwear

Specialist footwear is required in those activities which are weight-bearing, such as higher impact aerobics, running or step aerobics. Where activities are non-weight-bearing or low-impact, such as steady but not extremely brisk walking, cycling, rowing, stepping machine exercising, then a soft-soled shoe with laces is suitable. In the early stages of beginning an exercise or activity programme it is likely that a specialist shoe will not have to be purchased and that the client already possesses something suitable. Once a client progresses to a level where more cushioning and stability are required, a good training shoe can be purchased for £30–40 ($50–60 US).

Poor posture and limb movement: summary of factors

In many of the activities described above, the importance of preventing too much forward flexion of the spine or bending over was mentioned. It must be remembered that when an individual exerts themself to higher intensities, causing them to get out of breath, a natural reaction is to bend forwards. Bending forwards helps in catching one's breath, because in this position gravity provides an added external force to help expand the lungs and the rib cage. In acknowledging this phenomenom, it is important that the exercise intensity is set appropriately, as thoroughly decribed in Chapters 7 and 9, in order to prevent poor postures occurring in response to heavier breathing.

Poor posture and joint stress or pain thus occurs from: poor technique and coordination, wrongly adjusted seats or pedals on equipment, a physical weakness, a pre-existing joint problem, and possibly over-exertion.

Other health conditions which affect musculoskeletal function

Arthritis

When a person mentions they have arthritis, it is important to determine whether they have osteoarthritis or rheumatoid arthritis.

Osteoarthritis (OA)

This is typically associated with chronic and possibly abnormal wear and tear of the joint, of which every adult may suffer to some degree as the ageing process progresses. A previous injury which has altered the mechanics of a joint is also a possible cause of OA. In most cases, keeping joints mobile, without excess stress to them, can be beneficial in the long-term prevention of joint dysfunction and reduced mobility related to OA.

Rheumatoid arthritis (RA)

Medical advice should be sought prior to beginning or re-starting an exercise programme. It is common for people suffering with RA to go through phases where the joints are mobile, interspersed by periods of dysfunction, swelling and pain. If RA patients are cleared to participate in an activity, it may be a fact that a programme will have to start and stop from time to time. Keeping in contact with a client is thus important, to ensure that they return after a period of dysfunction is resolved.

In both OA and RA, it is typical that the problem will affect a client's ability to participate, but in many cases this should not be used as an excuse not to be active.

Strokes and head injury patients

The risk factors and corresponding health disorders for strokes (see Chapter 2) are very similar to those of coronary heart disease and thus the benefits may also be similar, as outlined in Chapter 11. With the input of an expert practitioner (specialist physiotherapist), it should be possible to adapt suitable programmes of exercise.

In both strokes and head injuries the full functioning of the nerves which stimulate and coordinate specific muscle groups can be impaired. The neurological impairment will thus affect strength, balance, and coordination to varying degrees and to specified parts of the body. Depending on the physiotherapist's recommendations, attempting to activate the traumatized muscles will require considerations for the pattern of the movement and with the aim to regain (if possible) some strength and coordination. Furthermore, patients' ability to understand instructions and put them into action may also be impaired. From the perspective of aiming to improve fitness and health adaptations in these individuals, this can be achieved by adapting exercise which first exploits the frequent activation of the unimpaired 'good' muscles. Non-weight-bearing activities, such as cycling or using recumbent cycles and possibly rowing machines, may provide the opportunity to monitor blood pressure and heart rate response in these patients. There may be the fact that even a low-level intensity of activity, which is of the correct movement pattern (as described by a physiotherapist), may well help stimulate improved balance or coordination in addition to the effects on the health of the blood and circulation. Finally, the psychological benefit to such patients, through the social interaction, sense of mastery and admiration of others attending the positive health-promoting environment of an exercise session/centre, can greatly restore self-esteem and confidence in these clients.

Identifying problematic limb movement patterns with musculoskeletal dysfunction

The correction of any unequal or asymmetrical actions is a key factor in reducing stresses and strains throughout the body. It may well be the case that there will be unavoidable asymmetries in muscle strength, length or range of movement in a limb, as is the case in an individual with a hip or knee replacement. In these situations, use of a non-weight-bearing bilateral exercise, such as on a rowing ergometer where the two legs perform the same action at the same time, will promote symmetrical movement. Use of a cycle or stepper machine is potentially beneficial in activating both limbs equally, but it must be performed with careful teaching to prevent excessive inequalities in the individual lower limb movements. Upper body torsions can be a good sign of unequal joint range of motion and muscle action imbalances in the lower limbs.

It is also important to consider that a client's cardiovascular fitness may physiologically allow them to work to a certain intensity, but if this is a pace which causes excessive strains, asymmetrical movements or imbalances in actions, the intensity must be lowered to a level where symmetrical movement can be performed. It may simply be a case of learning to perform the action correctly at a lower pace and gradually progressing to controlled balanced actions at higher intensities. There is also the problem that if an action is too slow, often typically found when using a treadmill or in swimming, the action may become awkward since there simply is not enough pace to invoke a rhythmical balanced pattern of movement. The exercise professional needs to optimize between exercise intensity and correct movement patterns.

Summary of limb movement with musculoskeletal dysfunction

The presence of a musculoskeletal problem is very rarely a reason for excluding people from beneficial cardiovascular aerobic activity and exercise. When such conditions are present, adaptations can be made to activities which either exclude the use of the affected joint without deactivating the rest of the body, or the activity is adapted to reduce the amount of stress on a particular joint, muscle or bone. Obviously, those activities which minimize or do not require the use of the affected joint should be exploited to the client's best advantage.

The body's position on a piece of exercise equipment, or during an exercise class, can greatly affect the amount of stress or poor posture throughout the spine, the pelvis and the legs. Excess protruding or poking forward of the neck will also cause inefficient compensatory action throughout the rest of the body. Strain and stress to the spine, pelvis and legs also includes the effects on the nerve fibres as well as the bone and joint cartilage, ligaments and muscle tendons.

11

Activity and exercise considerations for high blood pressure and heart disease

Hypertension and associated health problems
Effects of beta blockers: implications for exercise
Considerations for those with coronary heart disease
Chapter summary
References

It is very important to recognize that this chapter aims only to act as an introduction to considering exercise for people with high blood pressure (hypertension), stroke (CVA) and heart problems or coronary heart disease (CHD). Many of the elements on prescribing activity and exercise on hypertension tie in closely with the guidelines in Chapter 7. Except in severe cases, high blood pressure should not exclude people from participating in moderate activity or even more vigorous exercise,[1] once a pre-activity screening has been carried out by a doctor.

Concerning more severe cases of hypertension or with regards to CHD this chapter, unlike the rest of the book, is written only to provide the reader with a background to this topic area. If, or when, the time comes that the reader is more involved with these types of clients, this chapter will hopefully have provided an initial appreciation for the delivery of CHD exercise programmes. Further reading and certainly specialist training are required to work in the area of CHD exercise programmes and some of the recommended texts or guidelines recognized in this area (fully referenced at the end of the chapter) include:

- ACSM Position statement: Physical activity, physical fitness and hypertension,[1]
- ACSM Position statement: Exercise for patients with coronary artery disease,[2]
- British Association for Cardiac Rehabilitation guidelines,[3]
- Heart disease and rehabilitation,[4]
- American Association of Cardiovascular and Pulmonary Rehabilitation: Guidelines for cardiac rehabilitation.[5]

High blood pressure (hypertension)

The term 'hypertension' is used here to describe high blood pressure. Hypertension is caused by various biochemical/hormonal and physical reactions within the body that lead to the constriction of blood flow due to a physical narrowing (vasoconstriction) of the arteries. The term 'peripheral vascular resistance' is often used to describe this narrowing of blood vessels away from the heart, where there is an increased resistance of flow against which the heart has to pump. Peripheral vascular resistance can be caused by a number of factors including:

- an acute emotional response which leads to the release of hormones (e.g. adrenaline), where the restriction goes away once the emotional state is relieved,
- a very heavy maximal muscular contraction (e.g. lifting a very heavy weight, pushing a heavy object, shovelling heavy, wet snow), but once the muscle tension is released the vessels again dilate,
- more seriously, chronic problems which are acquired either by a poor lifestyle (e.g. smoking, stress, inactivity, poor diet, obesity), regular acute emotional bouts, or are inherited through a family history of the problem.

The exact measurement threshold (in mmHg, see Chapter 6) at which a person can be classified as being hypertensive may vary slightly from one country to the next or even from one doctor to the next. The general guideline for exercise professionals should obviously be more conservative than a for medical clinician. When the systolic pressure is greater than 140 mmHg and the diastolic greater than 90 mmHg, then this is the point at which concern should be expressed. If an exercise professional measures a client's resting blood pressure and it is above 140/90 mmHg, then:

- recheck it after 1 or 2 minutes simply to see if either a measurement error has been made or if it is affected by the client feeling anxious,
- if it is still raised, ask the client when they last had it checked,
- ask the client if their day to this point was particularly stressful or if they are a little anxious about attending an exercise consultation and having their blood pressure taken,
- state that as an exercise professional you are only able to use blood pressure as a means of screening and are unable to make any diagnosis; diplomatically recommend they first see their doctor to reassure them

Table 11.1 Classifications and ranges of blood pressure. (Adapted from Pollock and Schmidt[4])

Classification	Range (mmHg)
Normal BP	<135/85
High normal	130–139/85–89
Stage 1 (mild, borderline)	140–159/90–99
Stage 2 (moderate)	160–179/100–109
Stage 3 (severe)	>179/>109
Stage 4 (very severe)	Greater than above

that you and they require a more expert opinion. More often than not, the client will appreciate your recommendation to see the doctor.

A well-performed consultation should already have covered some of the above points prior to actually measuring the client's blood pressure. The best way to avoid any difficulties is to recommend clients see their doctor prior to attending the consultation. Recommending pre-activity visits to the doctor is especially important in those older than 35 years because, as noted later, this is when factors of age start to be linked with an increased incidence of hypertension.

If the raised blood pressure is borderline hypertension, as noted in Table 11.1, there is a chance that it may be due to the 'white coat' effect of attending the consultation; the doctor should endeavour to determine whether the raised blood pressure is an acute reaction or a chronic problem. People with healthy blood pressure who find themselves in a slight to moderate stressful situation should still have a resting blood pressure within the normal healthy range. If an exercise professional can establish a good rapport with a client's doctor, the situation may arise, as the authors have found, that if the client needs checks on their blood pressure the doctor is content to allow it to be taken at the exercise centre. This situation may be less stressful than having blood pressure taken at the doctor's practice, where people may perceive an environment more related to illness than wellness.

Hypertension and associated health problems

Hypertension is the major risk factor for CVA and is a primary risk factor for CHD, which is prevalent in 17% of adults in the USA.[6] Similar to the USA, a study in 1993 showed that approximately 20% of adults in England had high blood pressure (>159/94 mmHg).[7] A main fact for this book and a specific feature of this chapter is that hypertension has been shown to be reduced following the participation in regular activity.[1] Furthermore, it is closely linked to the onset of non-insulin-dependent diabetes mellitus/(NIDDM).[8,9]

Almost 10 000 people per year in England and Wales, between the ages of 35 and 64 years, die from hypertensive and cerebrovascular disease and it is the third most common cause of death after heart disease and cancer in women.[10]

Ranges for blood pressure

Hypertension has been categorized into various levels of severity and the higher the blood pressure level the greater the risk of developing the various conditions noted earlier (the levels are outlined in Table 11.1).

Many of the risk factors for hypertension can be modified, of which a majority are related to a person's lifestyle,[8] including:

- insulin resistance (see Chapter 2),
- obesity,
- diet (excess sodium intake),
- use of oral contraceptives,
- physical inactivity.

Some individuals, unfortunately, have risk factors which cannot be modified, including a family history of the problem, the process of ageing and one's race; there is an increased risk for people of Hispanic or African descent.[4,8]

There is increasing evidence that links obesity, NIDDM, hypertension and CHD when a person's body chemistry actually becomes resistant to the important function of insulin, but the mechanism for these links is not yet fully understood[8,9] (see Chapter 2 on insulin resistance). Such a problem is often apparent in overweight or obese individuals. Increasing physical activity, as discussed in Chapter 2, can reduce insulin resistance and if guidelines are followed, as outlined in Chapters 7–9, there is the possibility of a coincidental benefit to both NIDDM and hypertension.

Both shorter and longer term reductions in hypertension have been evidenced following regular activity and aerobic exercise.[11,12] Other research has shown that the benefits included a reduction in medication dosages following increased activity and aerobic exercise regimes.[1]

The American College of Sports Medicine (ACSM) 1993 position stand[1] on hypertension, which is a consolidation of research carried out on hypertension and exercise, makes the following recommendations:

1. Individuals who participate in endurance exercise will reduce the rise in blood pressure that occurs over time.
2. Reductions in blood pressure of 10 mmHg is evident in individuals with mild to moderate hypertension (140–180/90–105 mmHg.). Where 'secondary' hypertension is a result of kidney (renal) disease, even greater reductions in blood pressure have been shown.
3. The standard exercise regimen of 3–5, times per week for 20–60 minutes at the beneficial intensity recommended by the ACSM for healthy individuals is effective in reducing hypertension.[13] For those individuals who may not be willing or able to participate in exercise to the levels recommended in point 2 above, it has been found that activity intensities performed as low as 40% of VO_{2max} are in fact as beneficial, if not more so, as higher intensities (50–85% VO_{2max}).

4. Individuals with Stage 2 or 3 hypertension (>180/105 mmHg.) should undertake exercise training only after starting on drug therapy and guidance by a doctor. It has been found that this will enhance the hypertension-lowering effect of the drugs and allow a subsequent reduction in medication levels.

5. Following 30–45 minutes of moderate intensity exercise, systolic blood pressure can be reduced by 10–20 mmHg for 1–3 hours and in some cases this may persist for up to 9 hours.

6. Resistive exercise in the form of circuit training (>12 repetitions and lower weights) also has a beneficial effect, but higher resistance or pure muscle strength training does not appear to reduce hypertension. Most benefit occurs when resistive weights/circuit exercises are part of a balanced training programme which includes aerobic endurance exercise.

Like all benefits of exercise discussed throughout this book (health and/or fitness), the effects on reduced hypertension from activity only last if an active lifestyle is maintained.

Effects of medication

Although medication has a beneficial effect on lowering blood pressure, it is important to acknowledge that some drugs have side-effects which may actually interfere with important elements related to activity, including:

- cardiovascular responses to exercise,
- exercise performance,
- some of the health benefits associated with exercise.

Without going into any great detail of the numerous cardiovascular controlling medications, the one example used to illustrate the above points is the effect of beta blockers on exercise benefits and performance. Technically known as beta-adrenergic blocking agents, these are one of the most commonly prescribed drugs for reducing hypertension. They are also used in those who have heart disease, angina pectoris (chest pain from obstructed coronary artery vessels), or migraine, or those who have had heart attacks or coronary artery bypass surgery.

There are different types of beta-blocking agents, some of which may cause some or all of the side-effects to be discussed. It is therefore important to find out from the client the exact type of beta-blocking agent or other cardiovascular controlling medications they are taking, either through agreement with the doctor or by referring to a pharmaceutical formulary manual (see Table 11.2). In Britain, this manual is the BNF (British National Formulary); a local pharmacist will be able to inform you of how to obtain a copy.

The effects of beta blockers include:

- reducing heart rate by 20–40 bpm during both rest and during exercise[14] (see Chapter 6, Figure 6.10),

Table 11.2 Drugs commonly associated with treatment of CHD

Medication	Reason for prescription	Effect	Side-effects
Glyceryl trinitrate (GTN)	Relieves angina pain	Dilates coronary blood vessels increasing supply of oxygen	Headaches, may lower BP/dizziness Flushing, especially when warm
Isosorbide mono/dinitrate and other nitrates	Usually for angina Sometimes for heart failure	Vasodilatation	Headaches, flushing, dizziness
Atenolol (Tenormin) and other beta blockers	Treatment for angina and hypertension. Sometimes to prevent post heart attack damage Control of heart disease Atenolol sometimes given for lung problems as it acts mainly on heart, *not* rest of body	Lowers heart rate	Muscular aches, cold extremities, lethargy
Diltiazem (Tildiem, Adizem)	Treatment of angina and hypertension Reduces frequency of angina attacks, but does not relieve angina pain – too slow acting	Calcium channel blocker Interferes with conduction of signals in muscles of heart and blood vessels	Headache, nausea tiredness, dizziness
Amlodipine (Istin)	Treatment of angina and hypertension. Reduces frequency of attacks, but does not alleviate pain of an attack in progress – too slow acting	Calcium channel blocker Interferes with conduction of signals in the heart and blood vessels	Headache, nausea, ankle/leg swelling and flushing If tiredness and/or dizziness, should be referred to GP

Drug			
Digoxin (Lanoxin)	To slow heart rate and help regularity	Helps weakened heart to beat harder. Helping to remove extra water from the body improving symptoms such as ankle or leg swelling and shortness of breath	Usually only when dose too high Must see GP immediately if loss of appetite, nausea, vomiting, changes in eyesight, irregular or slow heart beat, weakness, confusion, drowsiness
Captopril (Acepril, Capoten) Enalapril (Innovace)	Used in treatment of hypertension and heart failure Not a cure, but a control	ACE inhibitors Dilate blood vessels, reducing force required from the heart to pump blood	Dizziness/lightheadedness, especially after first dose Above plus fainting may also occur when hot or when *exercising*, getting out of bed/chairs, etc. Alcohol can increase likelihood of side-effects Headaches, metallic/salty/reduced taste
Amiodarone, (Cordarone X)	To control rapid or irregular heart rate	Anti-arrhythmic agent	Metallic taste in mouth, increased sensitivity of skin to sunlight, greyish skin colour

- impairing maximal aerobic capacity ($\dot{V}O_{2max}$) through decreases in the heart's cardiac output and skeletal muscle blood flow.[15]
- suppressing fat metabolism at rest and during exercise by impairing the mobilization of free fatty acids in the blood[16,17] (see Figure 11.2, page 190),[16,17]
- increasing cholesterol levels and/or blunting the exercise training benefits on cholesterol,[4,18]
- causing increased breathing rate and breathing problems in some individuals during exercise through intiating spasm of the muscles controlling the bronchioles of the lungs (bronchospasm),[4,17]
- causing side-effects affecting mood (depression, fatigue, anxiety).[19]

Effects of beta blockers: implications for exercise

Effects on using heart rate as a means of predicting $\dot{V}O_{2max}$ or prescribing intensity

The heart rate reducing effects of beta blockers will obviously invalidate many of the protocols for predicting maximal exercise capacity (Chapters 6–8) which use an age-predicted maximal heart rate. These include any protocols which:

- predict $\dot{V}O_{2max}$ from a submaximal heart rate,
- use the age-predicted heart rate 220 minus age model,
- use the heart rate reserve method where a maximal heart rate is predicted from age.

The heart rate reserve method can, however, be used from a peak heart rate where an exercise test has been performed under beta-blocked conditions. This is often possible with cardiac patients who have undergone an exercise ECG stress test, where the peak heart rate or the heart rate at the point where the heart function starts to become abnormal can be used as the maximal heart rate[4] and entered into the formula in Table 7.1.

The two protocols in this book which remain independent of the heart rate effects from beta blockers are the RPE workrate/heart rate method thoroughly described in Chapter 7 and the Keele Lifestyle nomogram for predicting $\dot{V}O_{2max}$ from RPE and cycle workrate (Chapter 8). The Keele Lifestyle nomogram is at present under trials of validation and still requires some questions to be answered with regard to patients on beta blockers. The protocol in Chapter 7, however, allows for a target heart rate to be set even under beta-blocked conditions, but two precautions are required:

1. If the *dosage is ever changed* the client should be reassessed and the target heart rate must be reset.
2. *Noting the time of day when the medication is taken* in relation to when exercise is performed. It is important that the time interval between when the medication is taken and when the exercise session is

performed remains the same for each time a person exercises. For example, if the medication is always taken first thing in the morning and exercise was assessed and typically performed in the morning, the client's heart rate will be lower than if they were to exercise in the afternoon when some of the effects of the medication have worn off.

If the client's heart rate is found to be higher than expected, then ask:

- Have you remembered to take your medication today?
- Has your dosage changed recently?
- Did you take it at the usual time today?
- Is this a different time of day to when you usually exercise?

If the answer to any of these questions is yes, then the heart rate response will probably be different from that measured at the initial assessment.

The Brodie method for setting age-related target heart rate

This method overcomes the problem of beta blockers, or heart rate response, in unfit individuals or cardiac patients. Professor David Brodie, at the University of Liverpool, UK, has carried out research which was presented at the 1997 Dublin meeting of the Working Group on Cardiac Rehabilitation and Exercise Physiology of the European Society of Cardiology. He has adapted the very widely used target exercise heart rate zone chart which frequently appears on exercise centre walls, on aerobic equipment, in computer-generated exercise programmes (programmed into personal computers or exercise equipment), in exercise brochures and in exercise prescription guidelines and textbooks. The standard typical target heart rate zone was originally established with healthy, younger and more active individuals, and yet has possibly been wrongly applied across larger cross-sections of the population. Figure 11.1 clearly illustrates the adapted chart for cardiac patients or less fit beta-or non-beta-blocked individuals.[20] It highlights the optimal heart rate training zone and shows a lower heart rate peak than the traditional 220 minus age concept.

The impairment of $\dot{V}O_{2max}$ by beta blockers

There are a number of mechanisms which contribute to the reduction in $\dot{V}O_{2max}$ from taking beta blockers. The important fact from a practical perspective is that the client's exercise capacity will be reduced. If they have a previous history of being regularly active and subsequently have had to take beta blockers, then they should be informed of not being able to perform to the same levels (even submaximally) as in the past, although it is important to note that as a result of regular training the client can expect to have the same *relative or percentage improvement* in exercise performance as someone not on beta blockers.[21]

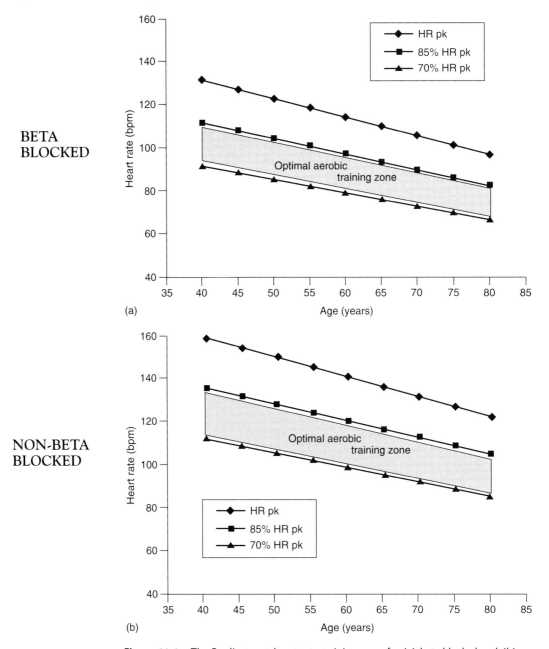

Figure 11.1 The Brodie target heart rate training zone for (a) beta-blocked and (b) non-beta-blocked clients and low fitness individuals. (From Brodie *et al.*,[20] with permission.)

Suppressing fat metabolism and possible increases in cholesterol

It is not uncommon for clients requiring exercise advice for health to have a combination or even all of the following three main CHD risk factors:

- overweight,
- high blood pressure
- raised cholesterol.

It is also not uncommon for the client's doctor to have recommended weight loss, healthier eating and increased physical activity as a means of combating the above risk factors. There is no doubt that beta blockers and increased activity can help reduce blood pressure as described earlier, but the client should be aware that the potential for the increased activity to help them with fat loss or improving cholesterol profile may be hampered by the beta blockers. It would thus be somewhat unfair for the doctor to expect the client to be highly successful in achieving fat-weight loss and reduced cholesterol from increased activity. It is therefore not unreasonable to get the client to ask their doctor to consider weighing up the priorities of risk factors (reducing blood pressure and fat-weight cholesterol, and increasing activity levels and/or fitness) and decide whether any alternative medication would be optimally more beneficial.

All is not lost, however, if the beta-blocked client can be encouraged to do very frequent activity, as illustrated in Figure 11.2, where Lamont et al.[17] demonstrated the comparison of fat metabolism (blood levels of mobilized free fatty acids) in beta- and non-beta blocked subjects before, during and after prolonged aerobic exercise. The main feature was that if exercise was prolonged for greater than 10 minutes, then free fatty acid concentrations in the blood and thus fat mobilization began to rise. In the beta-blocked group, free fatty acids rose above pre-exercising levels once the exercise was completed. The study confirmed previous research on how much beta blockers suppress fatty acid mobilization compared

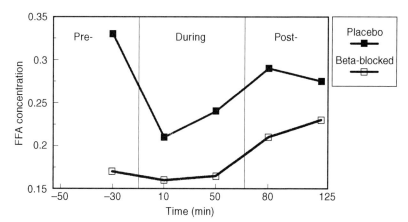

Figure 11.2 The effects of beta blockers on free fatty acid mobilization and fat metabolism before, during and after exercise. (From Lamont et al.,[17] with permission.)

with individuals not on beta blockers, but that there was much less difference in the levels between the two groups after exercise.

Considerations for those with coronary heart disease

As stated earlier, this section aims to give an appreciation of exercise considerations in this group of individuals and should not be used as a guide for establishing exercise and rehabilitation programmes.

In Chapter 2, the process of CHD was described as being caused through a build-up of a cholesterol and fatty based debris (atheroma) on the coronary artery walls, coupled with a degrading of the structure of the blood vessel wall at the site of the atheroma. The gradual build-up of an atheroma, in the process called atherosclerosis, can potentially cause a complete blockage of a coronary blood vessel resulting in a heart attack (see below).

A background to various conditions related to CHD and heart problems

Often commonly associated with CHD is the occurrence of a heart attack, technically known as a myocardial infarction and often colloquially referred to as either a coronary or an MI. The word 'myocardial' simply means muscle (myo) of the heart (cardial) and 'infarction' the death of a tissue. If a coronary artery is blocked, blood and oxygen are prevented from feeding that particular part of the heart's muscle and thus an infarction to that area proceeds. At the time of a heart attack there is usually a disruption to the normal electrical, chemical and mechanical functions of the heart, which in less severe cases is somewhat restored either naturally on its own or in more severe cases through cardiac massage, medications or electrical defribillation performed by a team of emergency clinicians. In the most severe cases this leads to severe dysfunction of the heart that can result in death.

In addition to those individuals who have had a myocardial infarction, there are various other CHD problems or heart conditions, which will be described more fully in subsections to follow and are often also included in rehabilitative or preventative exercise programmes, including:

- non-infarcted ischaemic heart disease and angina,
- percutaneous transluminal coronary angioplasty (PTCA or angioplasty for short),
- a coronary artery stent,
- coronary artery bypass grafting surgery (CABG or a bypass),
- chronic or congestive heart failure (CHF).

There are other heart problems not always related to CHD which also may be included as conditions benefiting from rehabilitative exercise:

- congenital (inherited) valve disorders leading to heart valve replacement,
- secondary valve disorders occurring from another disease (e.g. rheumatic fever in childhood or lung disease),
- in some cases total heart transplants.

Non-infarcted ischaemic heart disease and angina

This is where a person is diagnosed as having a partial blockage of one or more of the main coronary arteries, which has the potential to lead to complete blockage and thus myocardial infarction. Depending on the degree of the blockage and the corresponding severity of the condition, as determined by a variety of diagnostic procedures from ECG to nuclear X-ray imaging of the heart, a number of treatment possibilities can be implemented, including:

- blood thinning medication (e.g. heparin, aspirin),
- vasodilatory medication (e.g. beta blockers, ACE inhibitors and calcium channel blockers),
- clot-busting medication (e.g. streptokinase or altepase),
- cholesterol-lowering medication (e.g. simvastatin),
- possibly bypass, angioplasty or stent surgical procedures (see separate descriptions).

The term angina pectoris simply means chest pain which is typically associated with the blockage of an arterery or arteries surrounding the heart. Other conditions which often mimic very similar chest pain may include a hiatus hernia (a condition of the upper oesophagus) or pain referred from a strain or problem of the upper thoracic spine (between the shoulder blades). One medication typically used to relieve angina is nitroglycerine, which is usually administered as an oral spray or tablet under the tongue. This spray or tablet quickly dilates blood vessels and relieves pain related to CHD, thus acting as a means of identifying whether the angina was actually related to the heart. If the pain was not relieved from the spray or tablet it was probably due to other non-heart-related conditions, as noted above. It is important for people with CHD-related angina to carry their spray or tablets with them at all times, especially during activity or exercise.

Percutaneous transluminal coronary angioplasty (PTCA)

This is often simply known as an angioplasty and is a procedure used both as a prevention against myocardial infarction (MI) or as a means of secondary prevention against further infarction once an MI has occurred. The procedure is carried out with a surgical catheter (a very small flexible rod) entered into the body through the skin (*percutaneous*), and the catheter is moved down a blood vessel (*transluminal*) to a site and the coronary artery (*angio*) is reshaped or widened (*plasty*). Although based on an ingenious simple principle, the procedure is a very delicate operation, in which a tiny balloon at the end of the catheter is literally inflated (with a special solution and not by air) inside the narrowed part of the diseased coronary artery to widen it and restore a more normal level of blood flow through that section of the artery. Within 6 months of angioplasty being carried out, about 30% of cases, however, will suffer a renarrowing (restenosis) of the artery.[22]

A coronary artery stent

This is a 'scaffolding-like' structure, permanently inserted into the coronary artery to keep it widened, and serving the same purpose as an angioplasty.

A coronary artery bypass graft

This procedure, commonly associated with the term open heart surgery, has now become almost as common an operation as having one's appendix removed. It can be compared with the civil engineering procedure of building a bypass or express route(s) around a town because the traffic on the old roads through the town have become congested. The blood vessel which is used to to create the bypass is typically made up from a saphenous (long main) vein stripped from the leg.[22] Usually a patient will have more than just one constricted or blocked coronary artery, in which case multiple (triple or quadruple) bypasses will be performed.

Besides considering the functional cardiovascular benefits of exercise following bypass surgery (discussed later), consideration must also be given to the healing process of the leg, which has had a vein stripped from it, and the chest and shoulder girdle, which have been opened up to perform the surgery. The role of the cardiac nurse and the physiotherapist are important in these two areas. It is important that the leg is well healed, properly 'dressed' and protected and free of infection, which could be exacerbated by vigorous activity. With regards to the chest, it must be appreciated that the sternum (breast bone) has literally been sawn in half and the ribs and the shoulders have been prised backwards to open the chest cavity to perform the operation. Once the operation is complete, the sternum and then the skin of the chest must be sutured back together. In addition to the healing process of the sternum bone knitting back together and the skin healing, there is the possibility of the shoulders, neck and mid-spine area being strained, due to their being prised open and held in that position for the number of hours it took to perform the surgery.

The initial stages of activity rehabilitation should obviously question the prudence of vigorous activity which uses the upper body. However, from the authors' experience in working as part of a team, which includes nurses and physiotherapists, the use of a Concept II rowing machine has proved to be suitable and very beneficial in most patients 6 weeks after surgery. It is important to remember that before considering any mode of activity, it should be deemed suitable only after a thorough pre-activity assessment.

Chronic heart failure[22]

This is typically a problem which has occurred over time, where the heart has gradually losts its strength to properly pump out the blood to meet the demands of the body. It is not necessarily related to any particular malfunction of the heart muscle itself, except following severe myocardial infarction, but often arises due to the malfunction or disease of other structures including the heart valves that control the blood flow between the chambers and the heart walls (septa) which separate the chambers. It is also possible for a person with heart failure to subsequently suffer a myocardial infarction.

A defect in the valves or septa of the heart will disturb the normal pattern of flow of blood through the heart and the ability to create enough force to eject the blood from the heart to circulate the body. Subsequently there is an increased demand on the heart muscle to compensate for the abnormal or inadequate flow of blood which progressively leads to malfunction. One typical problem which can lead to the dysfunction of the valves or the septa is lung disease (including that related to smoking), which impairs the important flow of blood between the heart and lungs. Heart failure prevails because of the continual abnormal extra back-pressure against the valves and septa and extra work that the heart muscle has to perform to get enough blood through the lungs for the vital exchange of oxygen and carbon dioxide. With the 'failing heart' unable to get enough blood circulating, a cascade of peripheral problems also occur,[22] including

- poor circulation to the limbs,
- lack of oxygen and nutrition to the muscles and diaphragm,
- poor return of blood to the heart at the end of the circulation process,
- poor blood flow and nutrition to the vital organs (liver, kidneys, etc.).

In some cases the best care for heart failure is bed rest,[22] but in less severe, well-controlled chronic heart failure, low-level structured activity and exercise have been shown to improve fitness and daily functional capacity.[23] The mechanism for this improved fitness is due to the skeletal muscles, the diaphragm, and the muscles controlling the rib cage, becoming better able to extract oxygen from the blood and resulting in a lowered demand on the heart during a given activity. Although exercise in heart failure has been shown to improve functional fitness, there is little evidence to show that it may improve a person's long-term prognosis (future condition outcome). Alternatively, patients and their families may, however, regard a heightened quality and more active daily life in the mean time as being just as (if not more) important than the long-term prognosis.

Now that a brief description has been given of the types of conditions which may be considered within rehabilitative and preventitive exercise programmes, it is felt just as important to acknowledge some of the important aspects of providing and organising such programmes.

The rehabiltation process and exercise

A prime fact to acknowledge is, as evidenced in the previous section, that patients with CHD are not a homogeneous group[2] but a diverse group of people requiring very individual considerations. In addition to their primary condition, it is typical for them to have other problems which require consideration, including hypertension, lung disorders, diabetes, peripheral vascular disease and mood/mental health disorders.[2,4,24] These problems may have been the cause of the heart disease or have transpired, as with mood disorders, as a result of a heart attack.

The benefits of formalized exercise rehabilitation following CHD were first scientifically documented in the mid-1950s,[25,26] but one report often cited is the comment made by Heberden in 1772 to the Royal College of Physicians,[27] where he noticed that a heart patient who sawed wood for 30 minutes per day for 6 months was 'nearly cured'.

Following the onset of CHD which requires close clinical attention (i.e. hospital stay or surgery) there is a standardized procedure for rehabilitating and returning the patient back to a life which resembles that prior to the event. Standardized guidelines in the USA and Britain have established four individual phases or stages of rehabilitation:[3–5]

Phase I.   The hospital (in-patient) stay.
Phase II.   Early outpatient clinic or home-based care.
Phase III. Late outpatient community and home-based care.
Phase IV.   Community-based maintenance phase.

In each of the phases and relative to the individual patient's condition, the programme typically consists of activities of mobilization, physical activity/exercise, education, guidance, counselling and progression towards returning to improved levels of physical and social well-being.[3–5]

In phases I and II there is a greater focus on counselling and education, where the patients learn to:

- accept and cope with their disease,
- deal with the social (work or home) and emotional (stress, depression) problems created by the onset of CHD,
- become mobile and physically independent,
- take responsibility of caring for themselves, along with support from family or close friends,
- understand their medications,
- consider necessary lifestyle changes (diet, exercise, stress, smoking) in order to prevent future problems.

Phase III is about putting lifestyle changes into action, which includes embarking on a more structured regimen of exercise and activity, transferring the care to the family doctor and returning back to taking up previous responsibilities (at home or at work).

Phase IV is the end of rehabilitation and about maintaining the implementation of activities in phase III and living a healthier lifestyle as a means of preventing future problems.

Traditionally and still regarded in contemporary guidelines, the progression to phase III is recommended for 6–8 weeks after the event (heart attack or surgery). It has, however, been shown that in many patients with stable, less complicated conditions they have moved to phase III with structured exercise programmes 3 weeks post-event.[28–32] In fact, in these early progressions phases II and III have almost had to be combined.

The aims of cardiac rehabilitation

The traditional aims of cardiac rehabilitation are to facilitate the patient's return to an optimal level of physical, mental and social well-being.[3–5,33,34] Furthermore, because of the rapidly advancing techo-medical era in which we live, the justification for cardiac rehabilitation programmes is under increasing scrutiny. Such scrutiny is applied to its value with regard to:

- beneficial effects on prognosis (prevention of future complications),
- psychological and social well-being (the time, emotional and economic cost to the family, community and the country)
- the financial cost benefit to health service providers.

There is strong evidence to support all the factors listed above.

Improved prognosis

This has been demonstrated by:

- a 20–25% reduction in death (of all causes) in the 3 years following a person's heart attack,[35,36]
- improved exercise tolerance and functional fitness for healthy mobile daily living,[37–39]
- improved risk factor profile of blood pressure, blood lipids (fat and cholesterol) and fibrinogen.[40–43]

Improved psychological and social well-being

This has been demonstrated by:

- a sooner return to work and normal domestic life,[28,30,44]
- reduced anxiety and depression,[45,46]
- increased morale, self-confidence and psychological and social stability.[29,46–48]

Cost benefits

The financial benefits to hospitals have been demonstrated by the provision of cardiac rehabilitation programmes. The cost saving on average is about £100 ($160 US) per year per patient over the next 3 years, as compared with those who do not participate in an exercise rehabilitation programme, due to:

- a cost reduction from time saved caring for anxiety and depression,
- a reduction in re-hospitalization of patients
- the fact that when patients are re-hospitalized, the cost of their care is lower.[49–53]

More contemporary aims of cardiac rehabilation

Research since the the early 1990s has moved the agenda on from the earlier aims (during the 1950s–1980s), where the value of cardiac rehabilitation is now more than just a means of restoring physical functional capacity and reducing illness. It has moved towards emphasizing a progressive programme of risk factor reduction (hypertension, high cholesterol, smoking, inactivity) and achieving the earliest possible restoration to a 'productive' quality of life,[52,54] both of which have been strongly linked to a greater likelihood of future survival. After 12 months, however, the psychological and social levels of health between those who participated in rehabilitative exercise and those who did not shows little difference.[45,54] In spite of this longer term difference, the important element lies in the fact that an early return to a productive life is cost effective (socially, emotionally and/or financially) to the patient's family, their work and the community and to the health service providing care for that patient. The longer term cost effectiveness lies with preventing any further illness events through maintained risk factor reduction via a healthier lifestyle, which includes adjustments to diet, physical activity, smoking, etc.

The exercise rehabilitation programmes described earlier which started ≤3 weeks following a CHD event thus aim to implement the concept of the earliest return not just to health but to a productive life. Like the social and psychological long-term differences between exercise and non-exercise rehabilitated patients described above, it has also been common for the research to show little disparity in the physical and fitness benefits after 12 months. One of Britain's first and internationally cited studies by Carson et al.[37] is a prime illustration of the short-term and longer term differences between exercised and non-exercised post heart attack patients (see Figure 11.3). Unlike the social and psychological studies, however, is the fact that after 6 months there is usually a drop-off in patients continuing to participate in regular exercise. This problem may be related to an incorrect perception regarding exercise, since it may be thought of as a form of treatment that 'comes to an end' once the patient feels better (see Chapter 3). Those who have participated in a programme, even if it is less than 6–8 weeks, will have started on the path to adopting the appropriate activity behaviour and yet may not have been made aware of this fact. Once on this path, as described in Chapter 3, a client is more likely to continue for the rest of their life but only if the the right guidance and services are available.

Rehabilitation programmes are therefore as much about teaching healthy lifestyle behaviours as they are about affecting shorter term restoration to a productive life. As stated earlier, risk factor reduction of changeable factors (e.g. blood pressure, cholesterol, fibrinogen, mood, diabetes, obesity) created by physical activity and exercise only continues if the behaviour of regular activity and exercise continues.

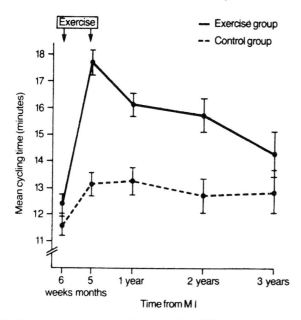

Figure 11.3 Fitness in post myocardial infarction (MI) patients, as assessed by mean cycling time. (From Carson et al.,[37] with permission.)

Lower level versus higher level intensity activity in cardiac patients

Lower intensity activity in cardiac patients is quantified in the same way as in healthy individuals, as defined in Chapters 4 and 7, where the effort requires using less than 50–60% of a person's $\dot{V}O_{2max}$. In healthy individuals working to levels of 65–80%, $\dot{V}O_{2max}$ is more beneficial from a fitness improvement perspective as compared to lower intensity activity (40–50% $\dot{V}O_{2max}$). In CHD patients, much of the research has shown, however, that lower intensity activity is as beneficial from a physical fitness perspective as higher intensity during the first 6 months following a heart attack.[28,55]

Changes leading to improved aerobic fitness (healthy versus CHD patients)

In Chapter 4 it was discussed that aerobic/cardiovascular fitness was a function of the strength and performance of the heart – the ability of the blood to carry oxygen and the muscles to take up and use oxygen. Factors related to the heart are termed 'central' and those related to circulation and muscle biochemical improvements are termed 'peripheral'. At this point the reader is reminded that the overall factor which limits the delivery of oxygen is central cardiac function and not the ability of muscles to take up oxygen which is made available to them.[39,56–58]

Following myocardial infarction, the cardiac muscle is impaired and thus a reduction in maximal aerobic capacity ($\dot{V}O_{2max}$; aerobic fitness) transpires. Intuitively, one may think that cardiac rehabilitation exercise will help reverse such an impairment of central cardiac function and lead to regaining fitness. Unfortunately, only in specific, more risky circumstances, where exercise in CHD patients is performed at high intensities (70–85% VO_{2max}) 3–4 times per week for >12 months,[59] is an improvement in central cardiac function found to be a means of improving fitness. Such an exercise regimen is not, however, typical of most cardiac exercise programmes, compared with those where putting patients at more risk through high-intensity exercise seems prudent and/or of any greater functional benefit to lower intensity exercise programmes. There is wide acceptance among researchers in cardiac exercise that any improvement in aerobic fitness in CHD patients is mainly due to peripheral factors such as the increased extraction of oxygen ability of skeletal muscles.[28,29,34,36] Such a fact is quite different to the fitness adaptations of healthy sedentary individuals who take up regular exercise, where improved fitness is clearly related to an improved central cardiac function (see Chapter 4).

Chapter summary

This chapter has highlighted some of the many important considerations for increasing activity and providing exercise programmes for individuals who suffer with either hypertension or CHD. In individuals with only hypertension, but no CHD, low-level intensity exercise appears to be as beneficial in reducing blood pressure as compared with higher intensity activities. There are also clear links between the coexistence of hypertension, diabetes (NIDDM), inactivity and the increased risk of future more serious CHD.

Guidelines for providing exercise for patients following hospital-based treatment for CHD includes four different phases of a programme. The four phases start with in-patient mobility activities, following on to structured exercise programmes and encouraging and guiding patients towards adopting a lifelong behaviour of physical activity. It appears that the earlier patients can begin their rehabilitation programme, which is sometimes as early as 2–3 weeks following myocardial infarction or surgery, the more effective the results will be physically, socially and psychologically for the patients and more cost effective for the health service providers. It appears that, unlike healthy individuals, safer lower intensity level activities are as beneficial to improving aerobic fitness in CHD patients as higher intensity activities. Furthermore, improvements in aerobic fitness in CHD patients, unlike in healthy sedentary individuals, are mainly due to peripheral skeletal muscle and circulation adaptations and not central cardiac adaptations.

References

1. American College of Sports Medicine (1993) Position Stand: Physical activity, physical fitness, and hypertension. *Med. Sci. Sports Exerc.*, **25**(10), i–x.

2. American College of Sports Medicine (1994) Position stand: Exercise for patients with coronary artery disease. *Med. Sci. Sports Exerc.*, **26**(3), i–v.

3. Coats, A., McGee, H., Stokes, H. and Thompson, D. (1995) *Guidelines for Cardiac Rehabilitation*. The British Association for Cardiac Rehabilitation/ Blackwell Science, Oxford.

4. Pollock M. and Schmidt, D. (1995) *Heart Disease and Rehabilitation*, Human Kinetics, Champaign Il.

5. Guidelines for cardiac rehabilitation programmes (1995) American Association for Cardiovascular and Pulmonary Rehabilitation/Human Kinetics, Champaign, Il.

6. Rowland, M. and Roberts, J. (1982). *NCHS Advance Data*, No. 84, 8 October, Vital and Health Statistics of the Center for Health Statistics, U.S. Department of Health and Human Services.

7. Bennet N. (1993) *Health Survey for England*, Department of Health, London.

8. Wilmore, J.H. and Costill, D.L. (1994) *Physiology of Sport and Exercise*, Human Kinetics, Champaign, Il.

9. Helmrich, S.P., Ragland, D.R. and Paffenbarger, R.S. (1994) Prevention of non-insulin-dependent diabetes mellitis with physical activity. *Med. Sci. Sports Exerc.*, **26**, 824–830.

10. Office of Population Census and Surveys (1992) In *Health Update 5*, OPCS, London.

11. Paffenbarger, R.S., Hyde, R.T., Wing, A.L. and Hsieh, C. (1986) Physical activity, all-cause mortality, and longevity of college alumni. *New Engl. J. Med.*, **314.** 605–613.

12. Lund-Johansen, P. (1982) Physical activity and hypertension. *Scand. J. Soc. Med.*, **S29**, 185–194.

13. American College of Sports Medicine (1990) Position Stand: The recommended quantity and quality of exercise for developing and maintaining cardiorespiratory and muscular fitness in healthy adults. *Med. Sci. Sports Exerc.*, **22**, 265–274.

14. Davies, C.T. and Sargeant, A.J. (1979) The effects of atropine and practalol on the perception of exertion during treadmill exercise. *Ergonomics*, **22**, 1141–1146.

15. Lundborg, P.H., Astrom, C., Bengtsson, C. *et al.* (1989) Effect of beta-adrenoreceptor blockade on exercise performance and metabolism. *Clin. Sci.*, **61**, 299–305.

16. Kaiser, P. (1987) Physical performance and muscle metabolism during beta-adrenergic blockade in man. *Acta Physiol. Scand.* (suppl)., **536**, 1–44.

17. Lamont, L.S., Romito, R., Finkelhor, R.S. and Kalhan, S.C. (1997) Beta-1-adrenoreceptors regulate resting metabolic rate. *Med. Sci. Sports Exerc.*, **29**(6), 769–774.

18. Duncan, J.J., Vandrager, H., Farr, J.E. *et al.* (1989) Effect of intrinsic sympathomimetic activity on serum lipids during exercise training in hypertensive patients receiving chronic beta-blocker therapy. *J. Cardiopulmon. Rehabil.*, **9**, 110–114.

19. Patten, S. (1990) Propranolol and depression: evidence from anti-hypertension trials. *Canad. J. Psychiat.*, **35**, 257–259.

20. Brodie, D.A., Liu, X., Bundred, P.E. and Odley, J.L. (1997) Age-related heart rate thresholds to optimise aerobic training in cardiac rehabilitation. In *New Insights in Cardiac Rehabilitation*, The European Society of Cardiology, Dublin.

21. Williams, M.A., Maresh, C.M., Esterbrooks, D.J. *et al.* (1985) Early exercise training in patients older than 65 years compared with that of younger

patients after acute myocardial infarction or coronary artery by-pass grafting. *Am. J. Cardiol.*, **55**, 263–266.

22. Kumar, P. and Clark, M. (1994) *Clinical Medicine*, 3rd ed, Bailliére Tindall, London

23. Demopoulos, L., Test, M., Zullo, G. *et al.* (1996). Low level physical training improves peak oxygen consumption in patients with congestive heart failure despite long term beta adrenergic blockade by enhancing vascular conductance and growth. *J. Am. Coll. Cardiol.*, **27**(2) (Suppl. A), 169A.

24. Morgan, W.P. (1997) *Physical Activity and Mental Health*, Taylor and Francis, Washington.

25. Hellerstein, H.K. and Ford, A.B. (1956) Rehabilitation of the cardiac patient. *J. Am. Med. Assoc.*, **164**, 225–231.

26. Gottheiner, V. (1968) Long range strenuous sports training for cardiac reconditioning and rehabilitation. *Am. J. Cardiol.*, **22**, 426–435.

27. Heberden, W. (1802) *Commentaries on the History and Cure of Disease*, T. Payne, London. In *Classics in Cardiology (1)* (Willins, F.A. and Keys, T.W., eds), Dover, New York, 196.

28. Goble, A.J., Hare, D.L., MacDonald, P.S. *et al.* (1991) Effect of early programmes of high and low intensity on physical performance after transmural acute myocardial infarction. *Br. Heart J.*, **65**, 126–131.

29. Debusk, R.F., Houston, N., Haskell, W. *et al.* (1979) Exercise training soon after myocardial infarction. *Am. J. Cardiol.*, **44**(7), 1223–1229.

30. Worcester, M., Hare, D.L., Oliver, G. *et al.* (1993) Early programmes of high and low intensity and quality of life after acute myocardial infarction. *Br. Med. J.*, **307**, 1244–1247.

31. Buckley, J. (1997) Rowing ergometer and treadmill exercise oxygen uptake 2 to 6 weeks post myocardial infarction. In *New Insights in Cardiac Rehabilitation and Exercise Physiology*, Proceedings of the European Society of Cardiology Dublin, May.

32. Buckley, J.P., Davis, J.S. and Mullis, R. (1998) Ratings of perceived exertion during rowing ergometer and treadmill exercise in 2 to 6 weeks after myocardial infarction. *J. Sports Sci.* **16**(1) 41–42.

33. Jette, D.U. and Downing, J. (1996) The relationship of cardiovascular and psychological impairments to the health status of patients enrolled in cardiac rehabilitation programmes. *Phys. Ther.*, **76**(2), 130–139.

34. Horgan, J., Bethell, H., Carson, P *et al.* (1992) Working party report on cardiac rehabilitation. *Br. Heart J.* **67**, 412–418.

35. Oldridge, N.B., Guyatt, G.H., Fischer, M.E. and Rimm, A.A. (1988) Cardiac rehabilitation after myocardial infarction: combined experience of randomised clinical trials. *J. Am. Med. Assoc.*, **260**, 945–950.

36. O'Connor, G.T., Buring, J.E., Yusuf, S. *et al.* (1989) An overview of randomised trials of rehabilitation with exercise after myocardial infarction. *Circulation*, **80**, 234–244.

37. Carson, P., Phillips, R, Lloyd, M. *et al.* (1982) Exercise after myocardial infarction: a controlled trial. *J. Roy. Coll Phys. Lond.*, **16**(3), 147–151.

38. Kavanagh, T., Shephard, R.J., Chrisholm, A.W. *et al.* (1979) Prognostic indexes for patients with ischaemic heart disease enrolled in an exercise centred rehabilitation programme. *Am. J. Cardiol.*, **44**, 1230–1240.

39. Shephard, R.J. (1988) Does cardiac rehabilitation after myocardial infarction favorably affect prognosis? *Physician Sports Med.*, **16**(6), 116–127.

40. Gordon, N.F., Scott, C.B. and Levine, B.D. (1996) Are blood pressure lowering effects of exercise training and dietary modification additive? *J. Am. Coll. Cardiol.*, **27**(2) (Suppl. A), 107A.

41. Fernhall, B., Milani, J., Gorman, P.A. and Paup, D.C. (1996) Fibrinolytic activity after maximal exercise in men with and without a history of myocardial infarction. *J. Am. Coll. Cardiol.*, **27**(2) (Suppl. A), 79A.

42. Schlierf, G., Schuler, G., Hambrecht, R. *et al.* (1995) Treatment of coronary heart disease by diet and exercise. *J. Cardiovasc. Pharmacol.*, **25** (Suppl. 4), S32–S34.

43. Sellier, P. (1995) Physical activity in the cardiac patient. *J. Cardiovasc. Pharmicol.*, **25** (Suppl. 1), S9–S14.

44. Bertie, J., King, A., Reed, N. *et al.* (1992) Benefits and weaknesses of cardiac rehabilitation programmes. *J. Coll. Phys. Lond.*, **26**(2), 147–151.

45. Stern, M.J., Gorman, A. and Kaslow, L. (1983) The group counselling versus exercise therapy study; a controlled intervention with subjects following myocardial infarction. *Arch. Intern. Med.*, **143**, 1719–1725.

46. Prosser, G., Carson, P., Phillips, R. *et al.* (1981) Morale in coronary patients following an exercise programme. *J. Psychomsom. Res.*, **26**(6), 587–593.

47. Ewart, C.K., Taylor, C.B., Reese, L.B. and DeBusk, R.F. (1983) Effects of early postmyocardial infarction testing on self perception and subsequent physical activity. *Am. J. Cardiol.*, **51**, 1077–1080.

48. Greif, H., Shulamith, K., Kaplinsky, E. *et al.* (1995) The effects of short term exercise on the cognitive orientation for health and adjustment in myocardial infarction patients. *Behav. Med.* **21**, 75–85.

49. Levin, L., Perk, J. and Hedback, B. (1991) Cardiac rehabilitation – a cost analysis. *J. Intern. Med.*, **230**, 427–434.

50. Oldridge, N., Furlong, W., Feeney, D. *et al.* (1993) Economic evaluation of cardiac rehabilitation soon after myocardial infarction. *Am. J. Cardiol.*, **73**, 154–161.

51. Ades, P.A., Huang, D. and Weaver, S.O. (1992) Cardiac rehabilitation participation predicts lower rehospitalisation costs. *Am. Heart J.*, **123**, 916–921.

52. Haskell, W.L., Alderman, E.L., Fair, J.M. *et al.* (1994). Effects of intensive multiple risk factor reduction on coronary atherosclerosis and clinical cardiac events in men and women with coronary artery disease. The Stanford Coronary Risk Intervention Project (SCRIP). *Circulation*, **89**, 975–990.

53. Bondestam, E., Breikss, A. and Hartford, M.D. (1995) Effects of early rehabilitation on consumption of medical care during the first year after acute myocardial infarction in patients ⩾ 65 years of age. *Am. J. Cardiol.*, **75**, 767–771.

54. Oldridge, N., Guyatt, G., Jones, N. *et al.* (1991) Effects of quality of life with comprehensive rehabilitation after acute myocardial infarction. *Am. J. Cardiol.*, **67**, 1084–1089.

55. Blumenthal, J.A., Rejeski, J.W., Walsh-Riddle, M. *et al.* (1988) Comparison of high- and low-intensity exercise training soon after acute myocardial infarction. *Am. J. Cardiol.*, **61**, 26–30.

56. Saltin, B. (1988) Capacity of blood flow delivery to exercising skeletal muscle in humans. *Am. J. Cardiol.*, **62**, 30E–35E.

57. Davies, C.T.M. and Sargeant, A.J. (1974) Physiological responses to one and two legged exercise breathing air and 45% oxygen. *J. Appl. Physiol.*, **36**, 142–148.

58. Shephard R.J., Boulhel, E., Vandewalle, H. and Monod, H. (1988) Muscle mass as a factor limiting physical work. *J. Appl. Physiol.*, **64**, 1472–1479.

59. Ehsani, A.A., Heath, G., Hagberg, J.M. *et al.* (1981) Effects of 12 months of intense exercise training on ischaemic ST segment depression in patients with coronary artery disease. *Circulation*, **64**(6), 1116–1124.

12
Health and exercise consultations

Measurements and changes
Setting the scene for the consultation
The consultation process
Part A. The subjective psychological, social and medical history
Part B. The aims of the exercise programme for the client
Part C. Objective health and fitness measures
Part D. Cardiovascular fitness and the exercise programmes and prescription
References

The importance of this chapter is that it is about carrying out a health and exercise consultation and not solely a fitness assessment or test. The word 'consultation' in the dictionary and thesaurus is synonymous with such terms as talk, conference, discussion, chat, communication, counsel, dialogue, deliberation and confabulation. With regards to the health and exercise consultation, it is all of these things relating to the individual health, activity, exercise and fitness needs of the client.

Measurements and changes

What is important to the client?
What is important to the exercise professional?
Whose means of measuring are more important, the client's own ways of evaluating their improvement and benefits or the exercise professional's technical physiological measures?
When are the exercise professional's physiological measures important?

If measurement of various physical parameters (e.g. height, weight, body composition, flexibility, strength and cardiovascular stamina) can be applied as an effective component in consulting with the client towards serving their needs, then there is no question of their value. However, training programmes for health and exercise consultants have traditionally focused more on the testing of specific health and fitness parameters. Such a focus has typically led to telling the client how *poor*, *average*, *good* or *excellent* they are in relation to the population, as opposed to acknowledging the underlying factors which affect participation. With this book focusing on health-based activity and delivering programmes for the more sedentary, older individuals, or clients with odd aches, pains or ailments, many of the typical measurements may be less valid because they have been derived from more athletic populations.

It is almost a certainty, as highlighted in Chapter 2, that since 70–80% of the populations of Britain and the USA are sedentary and 50–60% of these populations are overweight, a traditional fitness assessment will just confirm what many clients already know prior to arriving for their appointment – *they are overweight and have little stamina*. It is for this reason that the reader may be disappointed to find no table of norms in this book which gives ratings of where an individual may stand in relation to others on weight, body composition, flexibility, strength and cardiovascular stamina. It is not that the authors think that norm tables are wholly redundant, but that two facts should be acknowledged:

- this text concentrates on what to do with measures, once they have been taken (e.g. $\dot{V}O_{2max}$ in Chapter 9), as tools for *prescription* as opposed to tools for *description* which often negatively confirms a point the client already knows,
- they are widely available in books, leaflets and texts, and are provided in practically every exercise consultant's training course package that has ever been given.

Possibly more important with regard to the consultation process is assessing the various physical health, psychological and social elements which either enhance or restrict the clients ability to perform regular activity. In Chapter 3 the barriers to activity covered many of these factors. Within these measures and during the consultation, the exercise professional should seek to find out what measures and benefits the client feels are important to them, in their own words, as a result of participating. It is extremely important to write these comments down, even though some of them may seem unreasonable or invalid. Making a note of any unattainable, invalid or misconceived aims will allow discussions for the future, where possibly telling the client, at first, that they have some misconceptions could seem abrupt and deter other important elements of the consultation. Over the course of a consultation a client will make some remarks which may be related to the aims important to them, such as:

- 'I'd like to to go down to the next dress size if I could'.
- 'I'd like to get into my jeans I bought last summer before I had my baby'.

- 'I'd like not to get out of puff, when walking the grand-children home from school'.
- 'I'd like to have more energy when I get home from work, so I can enjoy working in the garden more'.
- 'I'd like to feel more alert at my new job, which at the moment is tiring and stressful'.
- 'I'd like to feel more toned in my bum, tum, hips and thighs'.
- 'I feel overweight and tired since having my hysterectomy'.
- 'I have put on 7 or 8 pounds since stopping smoking'.
- 'I feel aches and stiffness when I get up in the morning'.
- 'I haven't been sleeping very well the last few months'.
- 'Now that I'm retired I want to feel I can play golf 3 or 4 times a week'.
- 'My neck and back have been feeling a bit stiff when playing tennis'.

These are actual comments which have been made by clients. After the client has been active or exercising for a few months, it is much more valid to them to ask whether they have noticed any change in these feelings or comments as compared to attempting to describe the change in some physiological terminology. Furthermore, clients are often surprised that the exercise professional has actually taken note of such their comments. It is much more important, for example, that a person knows they have gone down a dress size, get less out of puff when walking up a hill, comment they feel more alert and are sleeping better, than for some exercise consultant to tell them something that they do not necessarily understand, including: 'Your VO_{2max} has improved from 35 to 40; you have decreased your percentage body fat by 3%; you are able to reach an extra 3 cm; or your grip strength has improved by 7 kg. These measures are important for the exercise professional as a means of designing, adapting or progressing an activity programme to help the client, but should not necessarily be the main features for feedback. The obvious question from the average client if you give them objective physiological feedback in this manner will be: 'Is that a good improvement?' or 'What does that actually mean?'

Usually for improvements on these objective physiological scores to move into the next category on the population norm tables, where they move into possibly a lower risk category, will take a long time. The client may perceive only small improvements in physiological terms as not being very good. They must therefore be reminded of how long (years in most cases) it has taken them to get to their present state, and that it is quite unrealistic to think that they can turn their present condition around in a few months. What is important and keeps people motivated to keep active is when they have personal sensations of feeling good about themselves (the decreased waist size and fitting into their jeans, friends noticing that they look healthier and more toned, and feeling better mentally), even though in the shorter term their weight has not changed dramatically, or they are not significantly stronger or more flexible. In Chapter 2 it was stated that to gain a lasting protective effect against CHD by becoming more active from a long-term sedentary lifestyle, the turn-around time was similar to that for smoking – approximately 2 years.

Setting the scene for the consultation

Throughout the course of this book the authors have focused on how the individual may benefit both physiologically and psychologically from participating in cardiovascular exercise and physical activity. The message is always that the exercise must be relevant to the individual client's needs or desires. The client is likely to adhere more readily to specifically tailored advice and programmes than a general 'applicable to all' approach. A personal programme obviously allows the client to identify more closely with the programme if they can see that their particular circumstances have been considered. Chapters 7–9 provided the framework for setting personalized cardiovascular exercise programmes, while remembering that it was stated that the other elements of exercise and fitness (strength, muscular endurance and flexibility) were beyond the remit of this book.

An initial consultation is a useful first contact session for both the client and the exercise professional, where both parties can learn their mutual requirements and gain an understanding of each other's approach: a relationship can begin to be formed. This initial session should be used to build up trust and understanding between the parties, with the exercise professional taking the lead. A client may never have been in this situation before and the idea of being 'assessed' or 'tested' is probably perceived negatively by many people. After all, tests usually involve elements of pass or fail and assessments are usually compared with some type of 'norm' information. Quite naturally, this approach could in itself be perceived as a barrier to participation. From the outset or even before the client attends their appointment, it should be clearly stated that they will be attending a consultation and discussion session, which will also include some health and exercise measures to design a personalized programme. Evaluation of psychological and social readiness and physiological baseline information are part of this consultation process and are discussed in the next section.

There is a current debate between researchers, exercise providers and the health and fitness industry of what a valuable consultation should contain in terms of the balance between counselling, advice and physical measurements. The authors do not at this point wish to resolve such a matter, but hope to have provided enough information and tools in this text to allow the individual reader to make an informed decision for their own needs.

In the light of previous statements, by no means is this chapter meant to be a definitive explanation of the consultation process; rather it should be regarded as a framework based on both theory and experience. It should also be noted that performing an exercise consultation is an amalgamation of many skills, based on the application of a good working knowledge of exercise science, physical activity and human behaviour. It is essential that prior training has occurred. All too often it seems that the potential for making the change to a healthier lifestyle is prevented because of a bad experience in the initial consultation.

The skilled exercise professional must make a decision early in a consultation session about what is felt to be the most beneficial approach for that particular client and gaining the maximum amount of guidance information, without including anything which may be perceived negatively. This is obviously a difficult decision to make – a decision which may become easier with experience.

The consultation process

Before the consultation begins, the client should be properly introduced to the exercise professional, including knowing the exercise professional's name and title. Providing appointment cards and a leaflet of information to the client prior to attending can fulfil this criteria. There are four main parts to the health and exercise consultation; these are drafted out in the example consultation sheet in Figures 12.1(a) and 12.1(b):

A. Gaining subjective psychological, social, activity and medical history.
B. Consideration of the client's aims and objectives.
C. Taking objective health and fitness measures.
D. Give advice on activity and/or designing an exercise regime which considers points A to C above.

Although the following framework is set out into specific sections, the experienced exercise professional may find that at any time during the consultation the client will make remarks that do not necessarily follow in this order. Some client information may overlap into two different sections. For example, under the section of daily responsibilities the client may state 'I am a single mother with three children under the age of 10 and am having to work almost full-time', and under the medical section she could state that she is at present being treated for hypertension and depression. Furthermore, it may be appropriate to let the discussion flow freely, with the exercise professional prompting key points in order that information from all the sections has been gathered by the end of the consultation. Any of the sections can be expanded to suit the time availability or the level of service of which the exercise professional provides. Such sections on the relative importance of diet may come into this category, but caution must be taken to prevent spreading the consultation too wide where for physical, social or psychogical reasons the main focus of the consultation is activity and exercise.

Part A. The subjective psychological, social, activity and medical history

This section includes gaining information about what the client already knows or perceives about themselves, including their *name, date of birth, occupation, present and past exercise and sports experience, habits of smoking, alcohol and diet, medical history and musculoskeletal constraints.*

207

Name _____ Membership Start Date _____

Consultation Date				
DOB (age)				
Daily Responsibility/Occup **Desk, Driving, Stress**	Active [ ] Sedant [ ]			
Excercise/Activity History **Past 2 mth** **Past 12 mth** **Since Childhood**				
Social Behaviour **Alchohol** **Smoking** **Healthy Diet** **Awareness**				
Medical **Previous Chest Pain, High BP, Asthma, Heart Condition, Epilepsy, NIDDM** **Medications and related side effects** **Any family history of CHD Risk factors? (hi-BP, cholest., MI, stroke**				
Musculoskeletal **back, neck, shldr, hips, elbow, ankles, knees** **Clinically Diagnosed? Treated?** **Any other medical or physical problems we should be aware of?**				
Reasons, goals, aims of excercise needs				

G.P. _____ Informed Consent/Signature _____

Figure 12.1(a) A typical framework for a pre-activity and health lifestyle profile.

DATE OF ASSESSMENT:						
GENERAL PROFILE	Age Height Weight Blood Pressure Resting Heart Rate Flexibility					
PULMONARY FUNCTION	FVC FEV 1 EFFICIENCY					
BODY COMPO-SITION	Triceps Biceps Subscapular Suprailiac % Body Fat Lean Body Mass					
CARDIO-VASCULAR PERFORM.	VO$_2$ Max Target Heart Rate					

Test Date: _____ Time of Day: _____
Assessor: _____ Temp: _____

Time	W/load	H/Rate	RPE	B.P.
1				
2				
3				
4				
5				
6				

Test Date: _____ Time of Day: _____
Assessor: _____ Temp: _____

Time	W/load	H/Rate	RPE	B.P.
1				
2				
3				
4				
5				
6				

Test Date: _____ Time of Day: _____
Assessor: _____ Temp: _____

Time	W/load	H/Rate	RPE	B.P.
1				
2				
3				
4				
5				
6				

Test Date: _____ Time of Day: _____
Assessor: _____ Temp: _____

Time	W/load	H/Rate	RPE	B.P.
1				
2				
3				
4				
5				
6				

Figure 12.1(b) Typical objective measures taken during a health and fitness consultation.

Before embarking on the more official aspects of the consultation session it is important to gain an initial perception of how the person feels about attending the consultation and any apprehensions they may have. Opening questions should be aimed at allowing the client to put themselves at ease and may include:

- 'Have you ever attended something like this before?' If the answer is yes, 'How did you feel about it and was it valuable?'; if the answer is no, move on to the questions below.
- 'Do you have any initial worries or apprehensions about doing something like this.' A typical answer: 'It's taken me a few weeks to build up the courage to come and sign up, but I've just seen some other people of my age and shape in the gym, which makes me feel a little better.'

  Or
- 'Did you have any previous impressions of what it might be like attending a centre like this?' Answer: 'You usually think and worry about seeing people with big muscles or body-hugging outfits and people who seem to be very fit.'

There are numerous questions like these that the exercise professional can ask to get the client talking and many of the structured questions to follow will further provide the opportunity for the person to reflect upon their feelings, attitudes and expectations. Some clients will give very short and closed answers and others will give a never-ending history. What is important is that the exercise professional always guides the discussion towards the points which are relevant for designing a programme of activity or exercise which provides a foundation for long-term participation.

One last question which should always be asked prior to taking any official notes is 'Are you aware of what happens in a consultation like this?' The exercise professional should state for example: 'In order for me to help set you an appropriate activity or exercise regimen, I need to obtain some information about your health, your aims and time availability and then make some basic health checks of blood pressure, height and weight. Depending on the information regarding your health and your aims, I may also measure your body composition, lung function and flexibility. One element, which I feel will be quite important, is to see how you respond to a steady pedal on the exercise cycle and monitoring your heart rate and using a scale of how hard you feel you are working (RPE), all of which will allow me to establish the correct pace or intensity of activity for getting you successfully started. All this information is taken and kept in the strictest confidence.

Personal profile

Name

It seems fairly obvious that the first item an exercise professional's records is the client's name, but this question also provides an opportunity to get their preferred or familiar title correct. They may wish to be called Mr or Mrs, particularly if they feel that there is a substantial age gap between themselves and the exercise professional. Alternatively, they may prefer a shortened version of their name or nickname, or they may be known by a completely different name. Addressing a person wrongly could annoy them and could present a barrier to establishing a rapport. Agreement on how a person wishes to be addressed or the use of a preferred name helps a relationship to be formed. Even better, if every time you see them you remember their name, they will hold you in a higher regard.

Date of birth

Establishing the age of the client may be a fairly sensitive issue. Often asking a person 'What is your age?' can be perceived as being rude or embarrassing. It is more professional to ask a person their date of birth. This also allows the exercise professional to know whether the client is closer in months or days to their subsequent year or to their present age. One's age is also required in many of the exercise prescription parameters, especially when heart rate is to be considered.

Knowing a person's age can sometimes give insight into people's perceptions, experiences and attitudes. For example, it may be difficult to physically discern the difference of someone born in 1923 as compared to someone born in 1933 or the same for two other individuals born in 1955 and 1965. From a physiological and health perspective there could be little difference. But the attitudes of someone born in 1923 may be strongly influenced by the fact of their suffering the social and domestic effects of World War II as a young adult, possibly even having to go off to war and fight. For the person who was born 10 years later, the war may not have had such an impact on them, and as a young adult they enjoyed the post-war pleasures and excitement of a rapidly developing and prosperous industrial era. The perceptions and attitudes of the person born in 1923 towards activity and physical fitness may be one of regimentation, whereas the person born in 1933 may have more of a carefree attitude and be less accepting and more questioning with regard to how and why they should exercise.

Occupational and domestic status and daily responsibilities

Understanding a client's occupational and domestic status provides clear information on:

- average daily amounts of energy expenditure,
- time availability,
- responsibilities,
- stress,
- socioeconomic status and attitudes.

Furthermore, a good analysis of a person's education, domestic and working life enables the exercise professional to pitch the level of dialogue appropriate to the client. There is nothing worse than either insulting someone's intelligence or completely baffling them with incomprehensible terminology. Having an idea of the daily experiences that the client encounters can be helpful in finding common ground for discussion between the client and the exercise professional, all of which creates a more relaxed environment and avenues for trust and rapport to develop.

Because the interaction between the client and the exercise professional is likely to occur on a regular basis, then knowledge of common interests allows the opportunity to ensure the client has a positive social experience, which can be a key factor in their long-term adherence. The exercise professional must, however, use discretion in how much familiarity they should develop with their clients because of factors of confidentiality and the collapse of what should be a completely professional relationship. Exercise professionals will, by the nature of the job, probably see clients or patients more frequently than any other type of health care practitioner or in fact any person providing a personal service. The exercise professional may also be a more prominent contact than the hairdresser or barber, the car mechanic, the doctor, the nurse, the 'therapist', the manicurist, the vicar or priest, the tennis coach, the golf pro, and the shop assistant. Possibly only the bartender or pub owner will be as much or more of a stable social professional contact for some clients.

In relation to CHD, the significant reduction in daily energy expenditure in people's lives since the 1950s, as noted in Chapter 2, is gaining more and more credence as one of the key risk factors. If a person's own objective is to lose weight through exercise, then it may be more than a case of just performing 2–3 hours of exercise per week. It may be important to identify where in the client's day they can simply be more on the move using their muscles and increasing circulation. As stated in Chapters 2 and 7, adding extra movement even at a low level during the course of one's normal daily occupation or responsibilities can certainly lead to far more calories expended. Though these calories will be expended in small amounts, when accumulated over the 14 waking hours of the day, they can easily add up to far more than those burned off weekly from an exercise programme. It should be explained to the client that an important fact about being fitter from their exercise programme is that it enables them to perform their daily routines with a little more vigour and this is possibly where the extra calories will be burned.

The executive that sits using the telephone all day in high-stress situations may need or want you to believe that they have no time for physical activity. Equally, a postal workers may suggest that they are active enough with all the walking or cycling performed to make the deliveries, and they certainly do expend considerably more energy than the executive or office-based worker. The aim for the postal workers might be to get them to develop more fitness-based strength and stamina, but for the office worker to simply increase activity levels, and participating to help relieve stress. In both cases there will be health benefits to be gained. Office and factory workers alike will often suggest that they get lots of exercise, by commenting. 'I'm on my feet all day', when in fact they may be standing still for long periods or walking intermittently.

Retired and unemployed people and anyone running a home (particularly if they have children) may also have pressures on their time, finances and accessibility to leisure facilities. These aspects need to be investigated and understood because they will probably be the main barriers to participation. Chapter 7 acknowledged the value of the types, intensities, frequencies and time available for a programme to be implemented. Finally, a conversation about occupation or domestic status again provides more opportunity for the client to talk about themselves, which helps put them at ease almost by distracting their attention away from the fact they are attending a consultation.

Exercise/activity history

Having some idea of the clients' current and previous activity experiences may give some insight into their exercise preferences, barriers and readiness to change. If the client has tended to favour group activity, it is likely that the social elements of exercise are important and enjoyable to them. Another common response is for the client to suggest that they do not get involved with any exercise, when in fact the exercise professional can create a positive point by stating that walking the children to school, walking the dog, gardening, home decorating and many other daily routines include physical activity and are beneficial. In other words, many people do not realize that they are already doing 'activity' to some degree and it may simply be the dose that needs adjusting for them to achieve health benefits and some of their personal goals. This observation can help the client feel more comfortable and confident about the idea of exercise.

Asking a client to recall the levels of activity they currently attain can be measured reasonably well using a variety of questionnaires and activity diaries[1,2] (Figure 12.2). There are, however, time implications for the exercise professional to consider in terms of balancing the usefulness of the information and the time it takes to analyse such information. These tools can, however, provide very useful baseline information for future comparisons.

Whether or not an individual is already participating in some exercise, this section allows a client's *training status* (see Chapter 5) to be determined, which will be valuable if or when applying the prescription intensities based on VO_{2max} given in Chapter 9. Is the person sedentary, moderately active, regularly or more highly trained and do they do their exercise for enjoyment in itself, for social reasons, or in training for another activity (e.g. winter skiing or summer hiking). Such questions obviously overlap with the later section on goals and aims. The volume and intensity of training over the past 2–3 months and then the past 12 months will help determine whether the client is moderately or highly trained and what intensity level they may prefer, as noted in Chapter 6 and 7 on the use of RPE.

Experience with sport and activity is another key element to this section. It gives information regarding when the client last participated in activity, exercise or sport and any attitudes, feelings or positive or negative perceptions they possess. The typical situation from the authors' experience is that many middle-aged people last participated regularly in sport or exercise at school, which is now more than 20 years ago. Negative perceptions may be held towards exercise because the person was not 'the sporty type' and was never very good at games, sports and the dreaded autumn/winter cross-country runs in the wind and the rain. As stated throughout this book, activity and exercise for health requires neither any great skill nor painful sensations.

The overwhelming success of individualized programmes lies in the fact that any competition is only compared with the client's original baseline. If this baseline is quite a low level of fitness, then they are assured to achieve much greater and more noticeable relative improvement than the already fit person. Many of the authors' clients have found a great deal of satisfaction as a result of an individualized programme which focuses on performance relative to themselves as opposed to

The Seven Day Recall (7 day par)

PAR#: 1 2 3 4 5 6 7 Participant_____

Interviewer_____Today is_____ Today's Date_____

1. Were you employed in the last seven days?   0. **No** (Skip to Q#4)   1. **Yes**

2. How many days of the last seven did you work?   ____ days

3. How many total hours did you work in the last seven days?   ____ hours last week

4. What two days do you consider your weekend days?   _____
                                                                                          (mark days below with a squiggle)

WORKSHEET   **DAYS**

		1 __	2 __	3 __	4 __	5 __	6 __	7 __
	SLEEP							
M O R N I N G	Moderate							
	Hard							
	Very Hard							
A F T E R N O O N	Moderate							
	Hard							
	Very Hard							
E V E N I N G	Moderate							
	Hard							
	Very Hard							
Total Min Per Day	**Strength:**	___	___	___	___	___	___	___
	Flexibility:	___	___	___	___	___	___	___

4a. Compared to your physical activity over the past three months, was last week's physical activity
    more, less or about the same?   1. More
                                                      2. Less
                                                      3. About the same

Worksheet Key:	Rounding: 10-22 min.=.25
An asterisk (*) denotes a work-related activity. A squiggly line through a column (day) denotes a weekend day.	23-37 min.=.50 38-52 min.=.75 53-1:07 hr/min. =1.0 1:08-1:22 hr/min.=1.25

Figure 12.2(a)   The seven-day activity recall questionnaire. (From Sallis *et al.*[2])

INTERVIEWER:

Please answer questions below and note any comments on interview.

5. Were there any problems with the 7-Day PAR interview?   0. No
                                                              1. Yes (If yes, please explain.)

   Explain any problems you had with this interview:

   _____

   _____

   _____

   _____

6. Do you think this was a valid 7-Day PAR interview?   0. No
                                                          1. Yes

7. Please list below any activities reported by the subject which you don't know how to classify.

   _____

   _____

   _____

   _____

8. Please provide any other comments you may have in the space below.

   _____

   _____

   _____

   _____

Figure 12.2(b)

competition with others. They never thought they would ever feel successful or get so much pleasure out of being more active – 20 or more years of bad feeling towards being uncoordinated and never really achieving any success at sport can be eradicated in just a few months.

Alcohol/smoking

It is up to the exercise professional to decide whether they want to use this information to either (a) remind the client that they are leading an unhealthy lifestyle and the future health consequences of such behaviour, or (b) simply take on board this information in a non-prejudicial manner as a means to gain more insight into the client. If the client later in the consultation states they are concerned about their weight, this gives the exercise professional the opportunity to state how fattening alcohol can be and considering cutting down may be as beneficial to the weight loss as the exercise. If the client consumes alcohol regularly at a pub, there may be some competition of leisure time between socializing at the pub and participating in activity or exercise. A compromise may be the best way forward, rather than a total replacement of one behaviour for the other. A great deal of caution has to be acknowledged when the client makes such bold and drastic goals as completely quitting one behaviour (going to the pub) and taking up another behaviour (going to the exercise centre). The heavier drinker has to overcome the hurdle of a psychological and social dependency, which again puts a strain on how time and desire can be restructured for activity and exercise participation.

Smoking, in terms of changing behaviour, is something which needs to be dealt with by trained professionals. Often a decision has been made where someone is aiming to cut down or stop smoking and wanting to take up exercise. In this situation a great deal of admiration and encouragment should be given by the exercise professional. Following smoking cessation, a majority of people will put on weight, and if the client is not initially aware of this, they may feel the exercise has failed them because it has not resulted in any weight loss. In fact, an exercise programme can play a part in preventing or at least reducing the typical amounts of weight gain which occur following smoking cessation. Providing support for people who have already made the decision to stop smoking is something the exercise professional can do as simply as stating 'Yes, you may put on weight as a result of stopping smoking, but how much more weight would you have gained if you hadn't taken up the exercise'. This can encourage the client to look at their exercise from a different perspective. Also, how well a person is able to sustain a non-smoking behaviour will probably reflect on their ability to change other health behaviours, including taking up more activity and exercise and adhering to it. The cost of purchasing 20 cigarettes per day over 12 months could quite easily pay for 2–3 years of membership fees at a typical health and exercise centre.

Medical history and medications

The first aim of this section is to find out if the client has any contraindications to exercise and if the condition(s) are at present under treatment or medication. Those clients under treatment or medication may perceive that the exercise professional is there to provide the comfort of a safe environment and that guidance is on hand at any time. In order not to approach this section too abruptly, first allow the client the opportunity to state any medical conditions they may have and then if necessary proceed to more specific questions on conditions which could be affected by exercise.

An opening question would simply be: 'Are there any medical conditions which you have that I should be made aware of and that could either affect your ability to perform physical activity or would jeopardize your safety or health while you are participating?' Some clients may respond like historians and leave no detail unremarked and others need some coaxing following this question. The important factor is that by the end of this section the person has made you aware whether or not they have at present or had in the past:

- any chest pain/angina, heart condition, high blood pressure, stroke or related surgery,
- diabetes and whether it is insulin-controlled or non-insulin-dependent,
- asthma and whether it is allergy or exertionally induced,
- epilepsy and, if so, how is it best to comfort or help you if you get an attack,

- dizziness, uncontrollable breathlessness or headaches from physical exertion or at any time,
- any other medical condition that could be at risk while performing exercise.

If the client has any of these conditions, have they been cleared by a doctor to participate in activity? If they have any medications which are used to treat these conditions, are there any side-effects (e.g. tiredness, weakness, weight gain or fluid retention, slowing or speeding of pulse rate) which may interefere with exercising? It is also important to acknowledge any medications which may hamper the benefits of exercise, which otherwise would occur if the client were not on medication. Post-menopausal women on hormone replacement therapy or those with thyroid problems on thyroxine may find that the medication has an overriding effect on their metabolism and thus interfere with the benefits of exercise on weight loss. In Chapter 11, the effects of beta blockers on physical performance, mood and fat metabolism were discussed. In addition to this are the medications which the client needs to carry with them at all times for relieving problems if they arise (e.g. nitrolingual spray for angina, Ventolin spray for asthma, glucose tablets or insulin for diabetes). Finally, the client asking the doctor about when to take medication on the day of exercising (before or after and how long before or after) could be an important factor in both psychological and physical abilities to participate with reasonable comfort and confidence.

It is advisable for exercise professionals to have a copy of the *British National Formulary* or similar publication available to them. This lists the effects and side-effects of most medications by generic and trade name. The client should be asked to identify all medications they receive, and the dosage and any side-effects which they experience. Understanding the medication and all its effects can help when setting an appropriate exercise programme

Any current medical condition should be reviewed and information provided to the client about how their exercise may have to be adapted to suit the condition or indeed how the exercise may aid recovery from the condition or help to reduce the symptoms (e.g. depression or high blood pressure). Some clients may feel that they do not know the exercise professional well enough to share all medical information with them. It must always be stressed that the professional practice of confidentiality will be applied. Surprisingly, sometimes a client may actually forget to mention even serious conditions, which may no longer be consciously considered by them to be a problem. In the authors' experience, some clients have actually not mentioned the following conditions when first asked during a consultation:

- past history of stroke,
- several myocardial infarctions,
- coronary artery bypass graft,
- serious motor control problems as the result of road traffic accidents and other traumatic head injuries,
- epilepsy,

- diabetes,
- musculoskeletal problems and injuries.

This illustrates the importance of offering a variety of lines of question in order to invite the *full* response. What you would consider to be important, the client may not. A professional but friendly tone should be adopted to encourage the client's confidence to talk openly.

A final question should always be asked: 'Are there any other health conditions I should be made aware of, which I have not asked about or you may have forgotten?' A signed consent by the client may also be advisable after this section is completed.

Family history

Collecting information about a client's family medical history of coronary heart disease and associated risk factors such as hypertension, diabetes and high cholesterol gives the client an opportunity to share any concerns they may have about their own health due to experiences within the family. It may highlight the fact that, in anticipation of the section on aims, goals and reasons for exercise, the client wants to avoid suffering similar problems to their parents, grandparents, aunts or uncles. The exercise professional can also ask questions around these concerns, such as 'So your father had high blood pressure – when did you last have your blood pressure measured?' If the response is 'It was measured as being a little bit high', the exercise professional can measure it. However, as stated in Chapter 11, a recommendation to visit the doctor may be required if it is near borderline hypertension.

Musculoskeletal problems

Chapter 10 covered much of the considerations on musculoskeletal problems. In the light of that chapter it must be remembered that the client is asked whether they have at present or have had any muscle or joint problems in their back, neck, hips, knees, ankles, feet, shoulders, elbows, wrists or hands.

Going through the list in this manner leaves no chance of omitting a problem. Also, qualify your question to find out whether a particular problem or injury was due to an accident, bump or bang (an extrinsic factor) or through an ailment/disease (e.g. osteoporosis, rheumatoid arthritis or a virus) or chronic 'over-use' or repetitive strain (an instrinsic factor). Has the client had any treatment, medication or surgery and are there any actions or movements which may exacerbate the condition. It might be wise to consult a physiotherapist who specializes in activity and exercise movement before choosing to prescribe specific modes or machines of exercise.

Part B. The aims of the exercise programme for the client

Establishing what the client wants or expects to achieve from exercise is absolutely central to devising any plan. The previous section on psychological, social and medical considerations may already have highlighted many aims without the client even realizing it. In knowing the client's psychological (e.g. motivation), social (e.g. time) and physical (e.g. medical, muscle or joint) constraints preceding this section, it can be determined how realistic the client's aims actually are. The physical assessments of heart rate, RPE and aerobic capacity will further qualify physical performance capabilities. It is very important to ensure that the client and the exercise professional are in agreement about the aims and goals, which will prevent two related factors:

- the client feeling that the exercise is not meeting their needs,
- the client not achieving their aims, resulting in dropout.

If the experience of exercise has resulted in not achieving the client's perceived needs, they may be somewhat reticent about ever trying again.

Understanding the client's aims

A sedentary individual may simply want to feel fitter, an obese person may want to lose weight, and a client with cardiac problems may want to return to a normal life. Understanding the client's own concept of exercise and fitness is a useful starting point (see Chapters 1 and 7). Also, attempting to know exactly what the client's aims are can be difficult; they may make overt comments but have some underlying ulterior (conscious or subconscious) motive. A man or woman may tell the exercise professional that they wish to lose weight. When asked if they feel overweight, it may become apparent that it is their partner's image of them that is giving this impression, but they would actually like to exercise to make more social contact now that the children are all at school or that their new job has a flexible timetable.

Initially stressing the need for *participation-based goals* (being active regularly) rather than specific *outcome goals* (losing weight, reducing stress) is suggested as being more appropriate. The exercise professional may discuss likely outcomes while stressing that the process of exercise will eventually lead to the outcomes if it is maintained. There may then be a need to discuss the client's goals and perceptions of how to achieve them, in some depth (e.g. looking at constraints of time, physical ability and motivation). Dispelling exercise misconceptions, myths and fallacies, as noted at the beginning of this chapter, may be appropriately discussed during this section of the consultation (see Chapter 3). In order for the exercise behaviour to develop, goals that are agreed with the client may carefully be set through progression, so that success can be achieved both physically, socially and psychologically. The goals of the client may change over time and therefore regular reassessment of the aims are required.

As stated earlier, recording the aims and comments of the client in their own words is an excellent way to relate changes or improvements in the future. Everyone uses language in their own way and will probably respond to positive feedback on their own words. The more contact and dialogue the exercise professional has with the client, the easier it is to relate ideas and advice which is meaningful to them.

Part C. Objective health and fitness measures

General profile

Blood pressure

It may be advisable to take blood presure as the first measure of the consultation. The client by this point is already seated and hopefully put at some ease now that a period of discussion has occurred from completing Parts A and B of the consultation above. Although Chapter 11 concerns hypertension and coronary heart disease, it also contains the underlying process of taking a person's blood pressure within a consultation. Furthermore, Chapter 11 provides the acceptable blood pressure ranges at which an exercise professional can except without first having a doctor's or nurse's measurement. As advised, it is best to have the clients see their family doctor prior to attending their appointment, which avoids the possibility of having to be the person to tell the client they may have high blood pressure. Chapter 11 clearly describes what to do if the exercise professional finds that a client unknowingly has high blood pressure.

Height/weight

Measurement of height and weight may be useful, as the exercise professional will need to know how heavy the client is in order to calculate/estimate relative aerobic capacity/VO_{2max} (if this is part of the consultation procedure) and to enable reasonably accurate setting of any weight-bearing activities (e.g. walking and running speeds, stepping machine resistance, aerobic step height). If it is decided that calculations of body composition (% body fat, body mass index; BMI) or lung function are to be assessed, then again height and weight will be required in these calculations.

Many clients may wish to lose weight as an outcome goal of their programme. It should be stressed that they are not being weighed purely for the purpose of future weight comparison. In fact, a sedentary less fit person may have a slight increase in muscle strength, even from aerobic exercise, which initially may cause a slight weight increase. In spite of an actual weight gain, however, it is likely that their body shape and physical appearance will actually change. A reducing waistline or neck size in this instance may occur before the scales show any weight loss and the client's focus is then switched from the number on the scales to tightness of their waistband or collar.

From the authors' personal experience is the case of a middle-aged woman that expressed her desperation at being 'so fat'. The scales were the only number that counted, and several 'weigh ins' per day were normal for her. Some education information and reassurance that the scales were not the most appropriate indicator of health status accompanied her exercise programme. Eight months later at a follow-up assessment she was asked if she knew her weight. She replied that she did not, but that she didn't care because she was now three dress sizes smaller. She was, in fact, almost exactly the same weight.

A person's weight is often a sensitive issue and the act of measuring a client's weight should be treated as such. Simply stated, it is as much required for setting the intensity of the programme (if not more important) than making any comparisons for the future.

Measuring height often prompts the client to assume that the exercise professional is seeking to categorize them on the basis of relative height to weight, perhaps by using a standard height and weight chart. If the client asks whether they are 'normal' height for their weight, it is perhaps useful to suggest that 'norm' charts are merely a guideline. In fact, body-builders who are heavily muscled could by the basis of these charts be categorized as overweight or even obese, when in fact they have very little body fat. This may be deflecting the issue, as perhaps the client is obviously obese, but if the point has been raised it is more than likely that the client realizes that they are obese. Merely confirming this for them may be negative, embarrassing and unnecessary.

Body composition

Body composition is any measure which gives an indication of the proportions of muscle, fat, water, bone and other tissues contributing to overall body weight. Too often this is based on just one simple instrument–measurement; the weighing scales.

There are only three things which a person can alter out of these components and these are muscle weight, fat weight and fluid levels, all of which can be affected by exercise. The daily and hourly change in an individual's weight is due to changes in body fluid (water) levels. In a typical steady exercise session (55–70% $\dot{V}O_{2max}$ for 30–40 minutes) it is quite easy to perspire away 0.5 litres of water, which is equivalent to 1 lb or 0.5 kg in weight. Many 'crash diets', which can create many pounds of weight loss, are simply a result of altering body chemistry and lowering fluid levels. To lose more than 3 lb (1.5 kg) of fat in less than two weeks is almost physiologically impossible. If such a weight loss does occur it is likely to be due to muscle or fluid loss. With all other things being equal, lost muscle mass in periods of less than a month only occurs if someone stops a regular muscular strength training programme or is involved in some form of starvation situation. The World Health Organisation recommend a total weight loss of about 3 lb every two weeks as being healthy. In fact a crash diet may force metabolism to slow down in order to protect the body's energy stores. Once the crash diet is finished, the individual returns to their pre-diet food and fluid consumption but with a slowed metabolism, and it is not surprising that they soon start to have a higher weight after one or two weeks than their pre-diet weight.

Typically, if an average height male is more than 180 lb (82 kg) and female greater than 135 lb (60 kg) they are considered to becoming overweight. The body mass index (BMI) is the means for making these judgements, because it is based on a ratio from height and weight. It is calculated as body mass in kilograms divided by height in metres squared (kg/m^2). The height squared provides an estimation of body surface area and thus it is assumed that body surface area is a function of body fat. Research, as outlined in Chapter 2, has shown that if this ratio is greater than a score of 30, there is a strong correlation with the prevalence or risk of developing diabetes, heart disease, stroke and high blood pressure. A score between 27 and 30 is classified in the overweight category but, as stated above, if this were a muscled body-builder, then they would be classed as overweight or even obese. This example show the pitfalls of this calculation. It is important, when using BMI, that body shape is acknowledged (see Chapter 2 regarding 'apple-shaped' and 'pear-shaped' physiques). Some of the issues in this area have already been mentioned in the previous section on body weight, but some form of body composition measurement is a usual part of most consultations.

A more valid form of body composition measurement is estimating or measuring the percentage of one's body fat (% body fat). Very rarely is % body fat measured in typical exercise centre situations; it requires either underwater weighing or some other sophisticated means that takes account of the weight of body water, muscle and other tissues. It must clearly be stated that most techniques are an estimation of % body fat. Practical means for estimating body fat now include the measurement of skinfolds, with more contemporary techniques using electrical impedance. Specific courses and manuals provide the methods for measuring skinfolds and then estimating % body fat. The YMCA's course is one of the most notable and their manual is called *Y's Way*. The use of skinfold calipers, however, can feel very daunting, intrusive and exposing to the client, especially if they are embarrassed and actually attempting to hide their fatness. It is therefore important to look at the pros and cons of such a measurement. Some alternatives, which are just as effective, to demonstrate fat loss following an exercise programme have been noted a number of times in Chapters 3 and 7 as well as below.

The above techniques for estimating (% body fat) have proved to be reasonably reliabe and valid, except in the cases where there is either an extremely fat or thin (low fat) individual. In measuring % body fat the feedback should focus on the amount of change and not necessarily using ideal or target scores based on norms, which just reinforce to some individuals that they have too much fat. Ideal or target scores often present too great a challenge to achieve, especially in those with high percentages (>30%) of body fat. The decrease in one's waist size or hip-to-waist ratio, which may not give an actual % body fat measure, can be as reliable (if not more so) and provides a very clear indication to the client that they have lost or decreased body fat, even when the scales show little or no change. The accuracy of two different people using skin calipers to measure the same person can be unreliable and the effective use of skinfold is a practised skill.

It is important to alter a person's perceptions gradually if they consider their weight or level of body fat as a measure of fitness. Simply showing a video of the London Marathon with competitors completing it in around $4\frac{1}{2}$ hours will quickly illustrate that people of all shapes and sizes can actually be fit. Again people must be reminded, as outlined in Chapter 2, that being more active and fitter is an independent factor for preventing CHD, even if people are overweight and smoke. It has been stated by Professor Claude Bouchard and his team that fatness is a genetic factor of between 25% and 40%. This still, however, leaves a minimum of 60% controllable by lifestyle factors.

Pulmonary (lung) function

Typical measures of lung function, including forced expiratory volume (FEV), FEV in one second (FEV_1), peak expiratory flow (PEF) and efficiency (FEV_1/FEV) are often included in standard fitness assessment programmes. As stated in Chapter 4, for most individuals lung function will not improve with fitness. In older individuals or those with chronic heart failure, as noted in Chapter 11, there may be some improvement with increased fitness. The explanation for why breathing improves with improved aerobic fitness, in spite of no change in lung function scores, is explained in Chapter 4, along with a quoted explanation of how to describe this factor to a client. Lung function in an assessment and consultation, and having it available for clients at any time, can be valuable for the following reasons:

- it is part of a health screening process which the exercise professional provides, and if a lower than normal score is recorded without prior knowledge by the client, then to have it further investigated by the doctor may prove valuable,
- if a client has asthma or another lung problem which needs checking from time to time, then that service is available at a venue which the client frequently visits,
- if the client has a baseline score taken in a healthy state, where a record is kept, and if for some reason they have to stop their exercise programme from an unforeseeable lung condition (e.g. chest infection, bronchitis, pneumonia), then the service can be available to check to see when their lungs have returned to normal,
- a record of a healthy baseline lung function may be welcomed by a doctor if for some unforeseen reason the client acquires a lung condition, because most doctors will not have a healthy baseline measure to compare with, unless the client has had problems in the past.

Part D. Cardiovascular fitness and the exercise programme and prescription

This final section to the consultation process literally brings this book full circle. Much of the focus of the book is about establishing the intensity, duration, frequency and mode of activity, with considerations of the client's physical and mental health and their goals and aims. Chapters 3–11 provide the means of designing activity lifestyle interventions or exercise programmes for better health. Referring back to Chapters 1 and 2 provides the rationale for why regular activity is so important for the improvement or at least maintenance of cardiovascular health.

References

1. American College of Sports Medicine (1997) A collection of physical activity questionnaires for health related research. *Med. Sci. Sports Exerc.*, **29** (suppl.), S1–S205.
2. Sallis, J.F., Haskell, W.L. and Wood, P.D. (1985) Physical activity assessment methodology in the five-city project. *Am. J. Epidemiol.*, **121**, 91–106.

Index

ACE inhibitors, 191
Activity choices, 115
Activity in daily living
   'activity points' accumulation, 123–4
   client advisory service, 123
   energy requirements, 128, 130
   exercise intensity equivalents, 130
   exercise prescription, 138–9
   initiatives for increasing activity, 120–1
   lifestyle activity intervention message, 119–20,
      121–3
   structuring intensity:
      for fitness/physical appearance, 126–7
      for moderate health gain, 124, 125
Activity history, 213–15
   seven-day activity recall questionnaire, 214,
      215
Activity, physical:
   beliefs/attitudes, 15–17
   cardiovascular health, 11–26
      risk reduction timescale, 14
   definitions, 1–2, 18
   'moderate' amounts, 5, 6
   thresholds for health/fitness benefits, 4–7
      recommendations, 18–19
Adaptation to exercise, 76, 77
   breathing responses, 84–8
   heart (pulse) rate, 85, 86–8
Addiction to exercise, 5, 8, 43–4, 46
Adenosine triphosphate (ATP), 80
   aerobic production, 81, 83
   anaerobic production, 81, 83
Adherence, 49, 50, 52
   long-term, 33, 34, 35, 38, 39, 49–50, 65
Aerobic exercise, 71–88
   anti-depressant effect, 36–7
   anxiolytic effect, 37

blood lipid profiles, 20
   health benefits, 5
   historical background, 71–5
   hypertension response, 182
   physiology, 75–88
   self-esteem improvement, 38
Aerobic metabolism, 75–88
   energy production, 80–3
   maximal aerobic capacity (V_{O2max}), 77–83
'Aerobics', 74, 75
   musculoskeletal problems, 174
Aerobics ergometers, 75
Aerobics exercise machines, 75
Affective (mood) disorders, 35, 36
Age, 212–13
   maximal aerobic capacity (V_{O2max}), 77
   maximal heart rate (HR_{max}), 103–4,
     105
   target heart rates (Brodie method), 187
Aims of client, 203–5, 219–20
Alcohol consumption, 215
Altitude, 77
Anaerobic energy production, 80–3
Anaerobic threshold, 84
Angina, 19, 190, 191
Angioplasty see Percutaneous transluminal
   coronary angioplasty (PTCA)
Anxiety, 36, 37, 45
Arthritis, 175–6
Asprin, 191
Asthma, 216, 217, 223
Astrand submaximal cycle test, 141, 142–7,
   152
Astrand-Ryhming nomogram, 143–4
Atheroma formation, 25, 190
Atherosclerotic heart disease, 20, 25, 26
Attitudes, 15–17, 24, 57–8

Attractiveness, 38

Back problems, 166–7, 169
Barriers to exercise/participation, 50, 54–7
    availability, 57
    emotional, 56
    lack of time, 55–6
    motivational, 56–7
Behavioural change, 57–66
    stages, 59, 65, 66, 139
        action, 62–3
        contemplation, 60–1
        maintenance, 63
        pre-contemplation, 59–60
        preparation, 61–2
        relapse, 63–5
        termination, 65
    stages of change (transtheoretical) model, 57,
        58
Behavioural cues, 51–2
Behavioural psychology, 32
Behavioural rewards, 52–4
Beliefs, 15–17, 57–8
Beta blockers, 130, 131, 137, 183, 186, 191, 217
    effects on fat metabolism, 189–90
    exercise intensity setting, 186, 187
    heart rate targets setting, 187, 188
    V_{O2max} impairment, 187
    V_{O2max} prediction, 186
Biological psychology, 32
Blood buffering system, 81
Blood doping, 80
Blood lipid profiles, 19, 20
Blood lipids, 19–20
    beta blocker effects, 189–90
    exercise response, 20
        moderate levels of activity, 18
    see also Cholesterol levels
Blood oxygen-carrying capacity, 80, 88
Blood pressure, 218, 220
    exercising, 112–13
    measurement, 112, 113, 180, 181, 182, 218
Body composition, 221–3
    modification
        exercise intensity, 158
        moderate levels of activity, 18
Body fat percentage measurement, 222
Body mass index (BMI), 23, 222
Bones see Musculoskeletal system

Borg scale, 105–6
Breath-by-breath respiratory analysis, 74
Breathing (ventilation) rate, 84–8
    adaptation to exercise training, 84, 85
    lactic acid accumulation, 81–2
British National Coaching Foundation (NCF)
        multi-stage fitness test, 142, 151–2
British Regional Heart Study, 18
Brodie heart rate targets setting, 187, 188
'Buddy' system, 48, 63
Bulimia nervosa, 36

Calcium channel blockers, 191
Canadian standarized test of fitness step test, 141,
        142, 151, 152
Carbohydrate metabolism, 81
Cardiac muscle function:
    improvement with exercise, 80, 87
    post-myocardial infarction, 197–8
Cardiac output, 87, 88
Cardiac rehabilitation, 193–8
    aerobic fitness improvement, 197–8
    aims, 195, 196
    cost benefits, 195
    exercise intensity, 197
    high-intensity exercise, 198
    prognosis improvement, 195
    psychosocial well-being improvement, 195
    standardized guidelines, 194–5
Cardiovascular aerobic endurance, 77
Cardiovascular controlling medication, 183, 184,
        185
    see also Beta blockers
Cardiovascular exercise assessment, 127
Cardiovascular risk factors, 11, 12–13, 181,
        182
    benefit of low intensity activity, 119
    cardiovascular rehabilitation aims, 196
    modification with exercise, 19–26
Cerebrovascular accident, 11, 217
    costs, 15
    exercise activities, 176–7
    exercise-associated health gains, 14–15
    mortality, 15, 16
    risk factors, 11, 12–13, 181
        exercise levels for modification, 17–18
Chester step test, 141, 142, 151, 152
Cholesterol levels, 4, 11, 19, 190
    beta blocker effects, 189

cardiac rehabilitation aims, 196
non-insulin-dependent diabetes mellitus, 21
see also Blood lipids
Client's aims, 203–5, 219–20
Cognitive functioning, 46
Cognitive psychology, 32
Communication techniques, 43
Competitive behaviours, 42
Compliance, 49
Concept II rowing ergometer test, 142, 152
Congenital heart disease, 190
Consent, 218
Consultation, 203–23
    activity prescription, 224
    client's aims, 203–5, 219–20
    initial session, 206–7
    objective health and fitness measures, 203–6,
        209, 220–3
    process, 207–23
        opening questions, 210–12
        personal profile, 208, 210–18
Contemplation stage, 60–1
Controlling own activity, 33, 34, 35
Cooper's 12-minute run field test, 141, 150,
    152
Coronary artery bypass graft, 190, 192, 217
Coronary artery stent, 190, 192
Coronary heart disease, 11, 179, 190–8, 218
    costs, 15
    exercise-associated health gains, 14–15
    medication, 184, 185, 191, 216, 217
    mortality, 15, 16
    risk factors, 11, 12–13, 181, 182
        exercise levels for modification, 17–18
Costs:
    affective (mood) disorders, 35–6
    cardiac rehabilitation, 195
    coronary heart disease, 15
    exercise activities, 42
Cues to exercise, 51–2
Cycle ergometry, 127
    energy expenditure, 128
    exercise intensity equivalents, 129, 130
    health-based exercise assessment, 127, 131
    musculoskeletal problems, 172–3
    workrate establishment from ratings of
        perceived exertion, 131–40
        data sheets, 133
        practical examples, 134–40

protocol, 132, 134
workrate/oxygen uptake relationship, 156,
    157

Depression, 36–7, 45
Diabetes mellitus, 11, 21–2, 216, 218
    type I (insulin-dependent), 21
    type II (non-insulin-dependent), 21, 23
        benefit from moderate levels of activity, 18
        coronary heart disease risk, 21, 22
        effects of exercises, 21–2
        hypertension association, 21, 22, 181, 182,
            198
        insulin resistance, 21
Dietary factors, 11
Distraction theory, 47
Domestic status, 211–12
Dopamine, 47
Douglas bag, 72, 73, 74
Dropout, 50
    activity intensity relationship, 117–18
    prevention, 62
Dropout rates, 50
Duration of activity, 116, 117

Eating disorders, 36
Efficacy expectations, 39, 40
Electrocardiograms (ECGs), 100, 101
Emotional arousal, 42–3
Emotional barriers, 56
Endorphin hypothesis, 46–7
Endurance ability, 77, 118
Epidemiology, 13–15
Epilepsy, 216, 217
Exercise:
    cardiovascular health gains, 11, 14–15
    cardiovascular risk factor modification, 14,
        19–26
    definitions, 1, 18
    health relationship, 4–5
    thresholds for health/fitness benefits, 4–7
    well-being relationship, 4–5
Exercise history, 213–15
    seven-day activity recall questionnaire, 214,
        215
Exercise intensity, 116–18, 130
    cardiac rehabilitation, 197
    cardiorespiratory fitness improvement, 159,
        161

charts for prescribing, 158, 159, 160
cycle ergometer, 156, 157
heart rate relationship, 130–1
limb movement pattern problems, 178
minimum threshold for benefit, 17–18
  beliefs/attitudes, 15, 16
protocol for individual determination, 132, 134
  exercise prescription, 138–9
  initial stages, 134–7
  progression of exercise programme, 138
ratings of perceived exertion relationship,
  130–1
rowing ergometer, 157, 159
setting with beta blockers, 186, 187
structured daily activity
  for fitness/physical appearance, 126–7
  for moderate health gain, 124, 125
training status, 117
trial and error determination, 117
walking/running pace, 155–6, 158
see also Workrate
Exercise intensity equivalents, 129
Exercise prescription, 115–40
activity in daily living, 138–9
consultation, 224
exercise intensity charts, 157–8, 160
heart rate targets, 131, 139
long-term adherence, 33, 34, 35
maximal aerobic capacity (V_{O2max}), 155–7
positive connotation, 33–4
protocol for individualized intensity determination, 139
  initial stages, 134–7
  progression of exercise programme, 138
psychological aspects, 33–4
ratings of perceived exertion, 131–40
training status, 155–7
Exercise response monitoring, 97–113
blood pressure, 112–13
heart rate, 97–104
ratings of perceived exertion, 104–11
Exercising blood pressure, 112–13
Extrinsic rewards, 52, 63

Family history, 218
Fat metabolism, 81
beta blocker effects, 189–90
Feedback, 43, 47–8
Fibrinogen levels, 11, 26

exercise effects, 26
smoking effects, 25, 26
Fitness:
adaptations, 76, 77
aerobic endurance, 77, 118
anti-depressant effects, 36
beliefs/attitudes, 15
definitions, 1
dimensions, 2–3, 76
health-related versus sports-related, 4, 18
levels of activity for improvement, 4–7, 157–8
metabolic, 3
Footwear, 175
Frequency of activity, 116, 117

Gender differences, 77
Genetic aspects, 12, 13, 91–2, 223
family history, 218
maximal aerobic capacity (V_{O2max}), 77
obesity, 23
Glucagon, 21
Gym weights equipment, 75

'Habit' of exercise, 49–66
Hand grip heart rate sensors, 102
Health:
adaptations, 76, 77
benefit from moderate levels of physical
  activity, 4–7, 18, 57
definitions, 1
exercise relationship, 4–5
Health belief model, 57
Health-based exercise assessment, 127
Health-related fitness, 4, 18
Heart attack see Myocardial infarction
Heart failure, 190, 192–3, 223
Heart rate, 81, 97–104
adaptation to exercise training, 85, 86–8
daily activity tasks intensity monitoring, 124,
  126
definition, 97
monitors and measurement, 98–102
nervous/electrical control, 88
oxygen consumption (V_{O2}) relationship, 103
ratings of perceived exertion, 106
response to exercise, 102–4
workrate relationship, 130, 131–2
see also Maximal heart rate (HR_{max})
Heart rate reserve method, 124, 125

Heart rate targets:
  exercise prescription, 131, 139
    initial stages, 137–8
    progression of exercise programme, 138
  ratings of perceived exertion during submaximal exercise cycle test, 131–40
  setting with beta blockers, 187, 188
Heart strength *see* Cardiac muscle function
Heart transplants, 190
Height measurement, 220–1
Heparin, 191
High-density lipoprotein cholesterol, 19, 20
  exercise effects, 20
  smoking effects, 25
Hormone replacement therapy, 217
Hypertension (high blood pressure), 4, 11, 22, 184–90
  ACSM recommendations, 182–3
  associated health problems, 181–2
  beta blockers, 183, 186, 187–90
  blood pressure measurement, 180, 181
  cardiac rehabilitation aims, 196
  exercise activities, 180–1, 198
  exercise effects, 182
  family history, 218
  modification with moderate levels of physical activity, 18
  modification of risk factors, 182
  non-insulin-dependent diabetes mellitus, 21, 22, 181, 182, 198
  obesity association, 23, 182

Insulin, 21
Insulin resistance, 21, 182
Intensity of exercise/activity *see* Exercise intensity
Intrinsic rewards, 52, 63
Ischaemic heart disease, 190, 191

Joints *see* Musculoskeletal system

Keele Lifestyle nomogram, 142, 148, 149, 152, 186

Lactic acid, 81
Life-style profile sheet, 200
Lifestyle activity intervention message, 119–20, 121–3
  'activity points' accumulation, 123–4

Limb movement pattern problems, 178
Long-term adherence, 33, 34, 35, 49–50, 65
  psychological aspects, 38, 39
Low intensity activity:
  duration, 117
  frequency, 117
  health benefit, 4–7, 18, 48, 57, 116, 119
Low-density lipoprotein cholesterol, 19–20

McArdle step test, 141, 151, 152
Maintenance of behavioural change, 63
Marathon running, 7, 8, 91, 223
Mastery, sense of, 48
Maximal aerobic capacity (V_{O2max}), 77–83
  absolute, 78, 79
  adaptation to exercise training, 84, 85, 86
  controlling factors, 77, 78
  definition, 77
  estimation/prediction protocols, 141–53
    comparative aspects, 152–3
  exercise prescription intensity (pace), 155–7
  genetic factors, 91–2
  incremental exercise cycle ergometer test, 86, 87
  modifiable physical factors, 78–80
  post-myocardial infarction, 197
  relative, 78, 79
  terms of expression, 78–9
  training status, 92–4
Maximal heart rate (HR_{max}), 103–4, 124, 125
  age relationship, 103–4, 105
  estimation, 104
Measures of health and fitness, 220–3
  blood pressure, 220
  body composition, 221–3
  height and weight, 220–1
  lung function, 223
Medical history, 216–18
Medication, 183, 184, 185, 216–18
Mental illness, 4, 36, 45
Mental well-being, 31, 35–49
  cardiac rehabilitation, 195
  mechanism of exercise effects, 46–9
Mitochondria, 80, 81, 88
Modelling, 42
Monoamine hypothesis, 47
Mood enhancement, 38
Motivation, 204

barriers, 56–7
  sense of mastery, 48
Movement ability, 163–4
Muscle fatigue, 81
Muscle oxygen extraction, 80, 88
Musculoskeletal pain, 165, 166
Musculoskeletal problems, 218
  limb movement patterns, 178
  overuse injury, 165, 218
  prevention in newcomer, 165–7, 175
    posture recommendations, 167
Musculoskeletal system, 163–79
  response to exercise, 164–5
    movement considerations, 168–9
  weight-bearing/non-weight-bearing activity,
    166
Myocardial infarction, 20, 60, 190, 217
Myoglobin, 80, 88

Neck problems, 166–7, 169
Negative outcomes, 5, 7, 52
  psychological aspects, 43–5
Nitroglycerine, 191
Non-weight-bearing activity, 166
Norepinephrine, 47

Obesity, 11, 12, 22–3
  body fat distribution, 23
  body mass index (BMI), 23
  effects of exercise, 23–4
  hypertension association, 23, 182
  non-insulin-dependent diabetes mellitus, 21,
    23
Objective health and fitness measures, 220–3
Occupational status, 211–12
Osteoarthritis, 176
Outcome expectations, 39, 40–1, 43, 219
Overtraining, 45
Overuse injury, 165, 218
Oxygen consumption (V_{O2}), 71
  cycle ergometer workrate, 156, 157
  heart rate relationship, 103
  maximal, 77–83
  ratings of perceived exertion, 106
  rowing ergometer pace, 157, 159
  walking/running pace, 155–6, 158

Pace, 155–7
Pacing, 118

Pain:
  lactic acid accumulation, 81
  musculoskeletal injury, 165, 166
Participant modelling, 42, 43
Participation, 31, 49
  activity history, 213
  barriers, 35
  self-efficacy goals, 43, 219
  self-esteem improvement, 38
Pennsylvania Alumni Health Study, 22
Percutaneous transluminal coronary angioplasty
    (PTCA), 191
Performance attainment, 41
Peripheral vascular disease, 22
Personal best (PB), 7
Personal challenge, 7, 8
Personal profile, 210–18
  record sheet, 208
Persuasion, 42
Phenomenological psychology, 32
Positive reinforcement, 43, 47–8, 63
  extrinsic rewards, 52, 63
  positive outcomes, 52
Post-exercise cool down, 81
Posture, 167
Pre-contemplation stage, 59–60
Preparation for change, 61–2
Prescription of exercise see Exercise prescription
Psychoanalytical psychology, 32
Psychological adjustment, 46
Psychological aspects, 31–66
  benefits, 34
    from moderate levels of activity, 18
  'habit' of exercise, 49–66
  impact of first sessions, 34–5
  musculoskeletal injury, 165
  negative, 43–5
  stress, 45–6
Psychology, 31, 32–5
Pulmonary (lung) function, 223
Pulse:
  monitors, 98, 99
  palpation, 98
  see also Heart rate
Pulse oximeter, 99

Ratings of perceived exertion (RPE), 50, 81,
    104–11
  Borg scale, 105–6

daily activity tasks intensity monitoring, 124, 126
  effective use, 106, 108
    practical aspects, 109–10
  estimation method, 111
  exercise prescription, 138, 139
    initial stages, 134–7
    progression of programme, 138
  mediators, 106, 107
  methods of application, 110–11
  preferred exertion method, 111
  production method, 111
  submaximal exercise cycle test, 131–40
  workrate relationship, 130, 131–2
Reference points for achievement, 42
Relapse to non-active state, 63–5
Respiratory analysis equipment, 72
Responses to exercise, 76–7
Rheumatoid arthritis, 176
Rockport 1-mile walk test, 141, 148, 152
Rowing, 169, 170
Rowing ergometer, 157, 159
Runner's high, 46
Running, 168–9

San Franciscan longshoremen study, 17
Second International Consensus Symposium on Physical Activity Fitness and Health, 22
Self-confidence, 39–40
Self-efficacy, 36, 39–43
  efficacy/outcome expectations, 39, 40–1, 43
  in exercise programmes, 41–3
    practical measures, 43
  theory, 39
Self-esteem, 7, 8, 36, 38, 204
  individualized activity programmes, 214–15
Serotonin, 47
Seven-day activity recall questionnaire, 214, 215
Short-term adherence, 49
Simvastatin, 191
Skinfold measurement, 222, 223
SMART mnemonic, 62
Smoking, 11, 12, 24–6
  attitudes, 24
  cardiac rehabilitation aims, 196
  cessation, 25–6, 216
    cardiovascular risk reduction, 14, 25
  effects of fibrinogen, 25, 26
Social interaction, 35, 46, 48

Sphygmomanometer, 112
  see also Blood pressure; Hypertension
Spiritual health, 4
Sports-related fitness, 4
Stages of change (transtheoretical) model, 57, 58
Step aerobics, 75
  musculoskeletal problems, 174–5
Step-ups, 170–2
Streptokinase, 191
Stress, 12, 45–6
Stress reduction, 37
Stroke see Cerebrovascular accident
Stroke volume, 87, 88
Swimming, 173–4

Talking threshold, 124
Technical instruction, 48
Temperature, 77
Theory of Planned Behaviour, 57
Theory of Reasoned Action, 57
Thermogenesis, 47
Thyroxin, 217
Time constraints, 55–6
Total cholesterol, 19, 20
Training programmes, 76
  maximal aerobic capacity (V_{O2max}), 77
  measureable responses, 76
  negative aspects, 5, 7
Training status, 91–4, 213
  exercise prescription intensity (pace), 155–7
  intensity of activity, 117
  maximal aerobic capacity (V_{O2max}), 92–4
Transtheoretical model (stages of change), 57, 58
Treadmill exercise stress test, 42
Triglycerides, 19

Valvular heart disease, 190
Variable resistance, 75
Ventilation rate see Breathing rate
Ventilatory threshold, 84
V_{O2max} see Maximal aerobic capacity

Waist:hip girth ratio, 23
Walking, 168–9
Walking pace conversions, 130
Weight, 4
  measurement, 220–1
Weight loss, 221–2

Weight-bearing activity, 166
Well-being, 2
    definitions, 1
    exercise relationship, 4–5
    see also Mental well-being
'White coat effect', 108, 181
Wireless chest strap personal heart rate monitor,
    101–2, 124

Workrate, 130–1
    submaximal exercise cycle test, 131–40
        datasheet, 133
        individualized intensity of activity examples,
            134–40
        prior health history screening, 133
        protocol, 132, 134
    see also Exercise intensity